The Politics of Change in the Health Service

Brian Salter

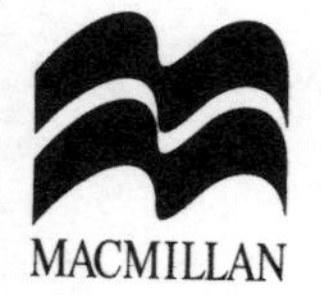

First published 1998 by
MACMILLAN PRESS LTD
Houndmills, Basingstoke, Hampshire RG21 6XS
and London
Companies and representatives
throughout the world

ISBN 0–333–65640–7
ISBN 0–333–65641–5

A catalogue record for this book is available
from the British Library.

This book is printed on paper suitable for recycling and made from fully managed and sustained forest sources.

10 9 8 7 6 5 4 3 2 1
07 06 05 04 03 02 01 00 99 98

Editing and origination by
Aardvark Editorial, Mendham, Suffolk

Printed in Hong Kong

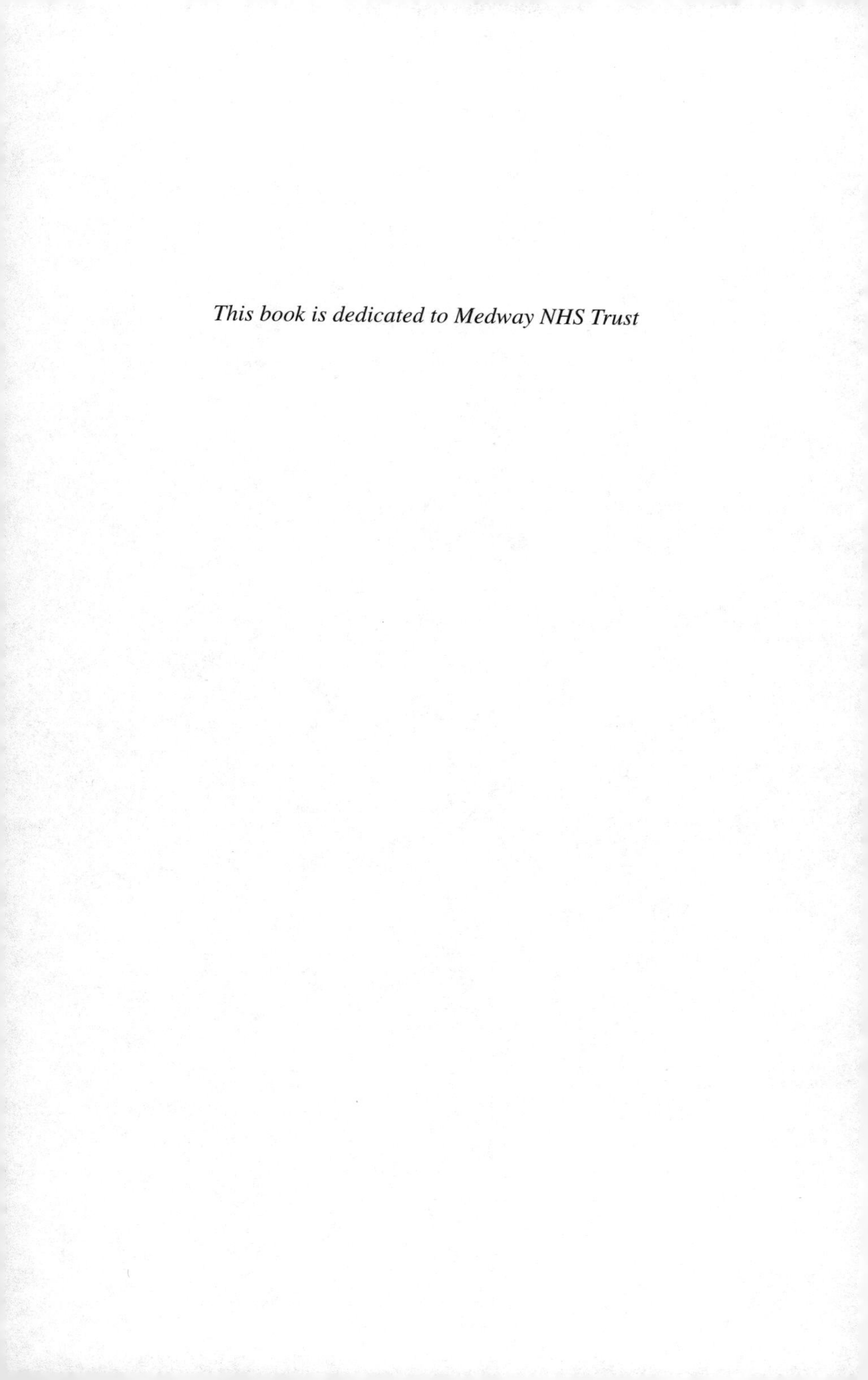

This book is dedicated to Medway NHS Trust

Contents

Foreword

No-one who works in the National Health Service can be unaware of the political pressures which permeate its daily life. Widely regarded as the most successful institution of the welfare state, the NHS is expected by the general public and politicians alike to deliver an ever-increasing range of services within a budget which has never been able to cover all the demands that are made upon it. Increasingly and, quite rightly, these expectations make their presence felt through clearer systems of accountability and public scrutiny which leave little room for manoeuvre, exposing for public examination and debate the NHS's failure to meet expectations whether they be realistic or not. It has a heavy cross to bear.

In a sense (and highlighted by my association with the writing of this book), this should not be regarded as surprising. The NHS is a public organisation which has statutory duties to deliver health care to the British people. Insofar as they perceive that these duties are not being delivered, they will legitimately demand that their elected representatives press for changes to be made. Thus politics and the NHS are rightly inseparable.

It has always been the task of managers and professionals alike (although sometimes in very different ways), to reconcile these increasing and often mutually exclusive demands and it is much more easily said than done. Traditionally there has been little filtering of public demand on the NHS and prioritisation, whatever form it takes, brings ethical problems (sometimes) and political difficulties (always). What is more, the effect of recent policy initiatives, including the separation of purchaser and provider functions, the Patient's Charter and the Health of the Nation initiative, has been to provide new and powerful vehicles for focusing the demands on the NHS – both old and new.

The arrival of the contract culture, perhaps more than any other factor, has provided a potent mechanism for identifying the NHS's success and its failures. Its performance, converted dispassionately into Finished Consultant Episodes and the like, is graphically displayed with the burgeoning power of information technology for judgement at a glance. In its wake, many health professionals have been left scratching their heads. What happened to the quest for quality? Is it to be measured or distorted by the imperative to deliver demanding contract volumes? What scope for a 'real' quality service, they ask, when driving to meet volume targets and when preparing for the close attentions of an ever-watchful media when the league tables are about to be published?

The main professional groups within the NHS are coming to terms with these changes in their own way. The doctors, it seems, having resisted the NHS reforms in their early years, are now 'getting on with the job'. For many this means a greater involvement with the non-clinical and the financial management of the service. General Practitioners have got to grips with Fundholding and many specialists have realised that the future of their trade in the NHS depends increasingly on their influence at least with the 'big purchasers' if not with all the little ones. After the early spats over the reforms it seems that the profession has accepted 'the new way' and the government and the NHS should be content with that.

For managers and for the nurses, some old and some new realities have had to be accepted. The managers have learned to wear 'the grey suit' and to recognise that while they will rarely be given credit for what the NHS achieves, they will frequently be the butt for all that goes wrong. That said, they are taking comfort from increasing recognition of their contribution from their professional colleagues and from a better informed public who know full well that large, complex and expensive organisations do not run themselves. For nurses, who remain the public's 'angels', there has been perhaps a more traumatic relegation of their status and influence at the top tables.

For both professions, it has become axiomatic that they must work within the dominance of medicine and that their objectives will rarely be achieved if they fly in the face of medical opinion. If the grey suits have few friends, if nurses remain the public's favourite, it is the medical profession's relationship with the government of the day that makes things happen – or not – in the NHS.

One of the key messages of this book is that all policy ambition must be set with reference to the reality of power structures and a recognition of the difference between rhetoric and practical possibility. In its development the work has engaged both managers and clinical professionals working in the Medway NHS Trust during a period of major transformation, with episodes of uncomfortable dialogue around the implementation of radical national policies and local structural change. Taking time out to contemplate the underlying power structures of the NHS does not fit easily with the pressures of daily life for managers and professionals in the NHS but is nevertheless an important aspect of their political development. This book provides powerful insights into these issues and they should not be ignored. To be oblivious to them is to stare through a glass busily but darkly, and with an increasing sense of frustration.

Ken Hesketh
Chief Executive, Medway NHS Trust

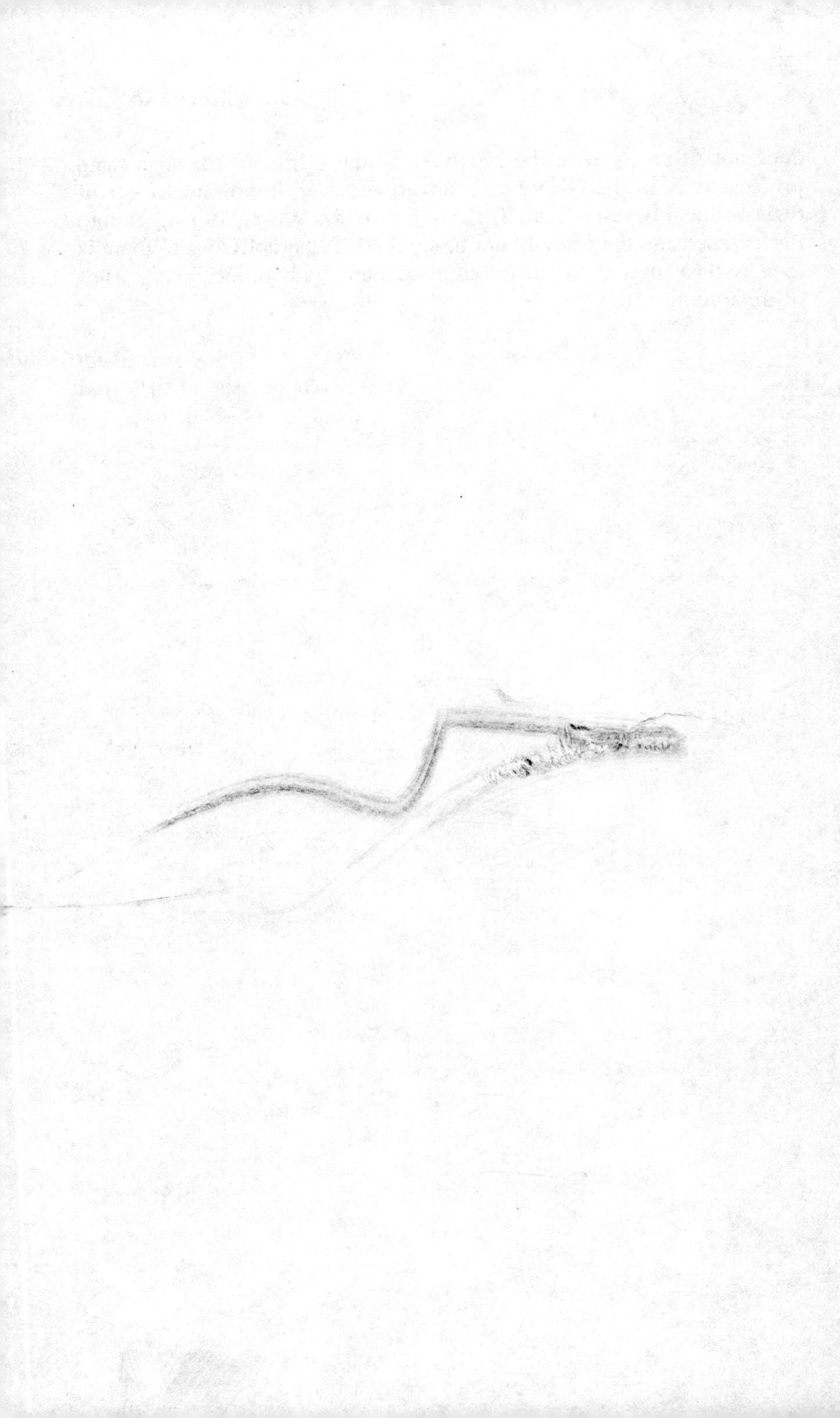

Introduction

As a political institution of the welfare state, the National Health Service has no parallel in terms of its resilience, its longevity and its abiding appeal to the citizens of the United Kingdom. Through its promise of free health care from the cradle to the grave, the NHS symbolises the essence of the welfare equation regarding the universal rights of citizens and the abolute duties of the state. Yet for exactly the same reason the Health Service also embraces the key political problem of an escalating demand for welfare which consistently outstrips the available state supply.

It is this problem, rooted as it is in the established idea of British citizenship, which acts to determine the balance of power in the NHS and drive the politics of change therein. Parties and their policies must, perforce, work within the parameters of the political problem and the hegemony of welfare state values that underpin it. To do otherwise is to risk alienating the support of those citizens on which electoral success depends. The Labour government can no more escape this fundamental truth than could its Conservative precedessors. Whether it will challenge the traditional values of the welfare state remains to be seen. But so long as those values and the concept of citizenship rights they embody remain dominant, so the political enigma of the NHS will remain to tempt and frustrate the policy makers.

In practice it is unlikely that the Labour government will initiate any dramatically new policies on the Health Service. There are three reasons for believing this. First, it is undoubtedly the case, as Klein observes, that 'the exhausting convulsions precipitated by *Working for Patients* have dampened the appetite for further change just as surely as the political and administrative labours involved in setting up the NHS inhibited a whole generation of policy makers from questioning its design' (Klein, 1995: 332). Second, if the 1991 reforms have achieved anything, it is the reaffirmation of medical power. Derived as it is from doctors' historic function since the foundation of the NHS of matching the demand for health care with the supply of taxpayers' resources from the state, this power has lately reached an accommodation with the new structures which it would be unwise to disturb overmuch.

Third, it is clear from Labour's policy statements on health that it has accepted the implications of these first two arguments; namely, that destabilising the system yet again is not an option. Its most important decision has been the retention of the division between purchaser and provider, from which much else flows. Contracts between Health Authorities and Trusts will be replaced by longer-term agreements; some form of representation will be introduced at Board level; and national and local targeting and monitoring will become more intense. Such minor organisational changes are unlikely to have any significant implications for the lessons of this book. GP Fundholders will be placed within an as yet unspecified system of GP commissioning (which will further reinforce their new-found power position) and the Labour Party has made it clear that the Private Finance Initiative will remain as a necessary source of NHS capital funds. The rhetoric will of course change, but not the substance.

This book is about the implementation of the reforms initiated by the NHS and Community Care Act 1990, and what that process tells us about political change in the NHS: its dynamic, its enduring laws and the inexorable subordination of policy to power relations. The theory and analysis employed are those of the political scientist and in the application of that theory the objective is to dissect and to understand, not to prescribe and evaluate. In this context policy assumes a contingent status. That is to say its significance is dependent upon its ability to impact on a health care system which is 'a political world in its own right, where the balance of power will determine the distribution of resources' (Klein, 1989: vi), and where the good intentions of the policy makers are of limited interest.

As the reader will soon become aware, the analysis is informed not only by the normal range of official publications (government and otherwise) but also by the detailed managerial and professional guidance which constitute the formal fabric of NHS life. Reading between the lines of this guidance is an exercise in textual criticism in its own right and can easily mislead the unwary. To test the validity of the ideas generated by the perusal of these sources, regular discussions were held with senior managers and professionals. Most of these informal sessions took place at Medway NHS Trust, where the author acted as adviser to the Trust Board. An important criterion in this exercise was the political utility of the analysis to the practitioners themselves: to what extent did it enable them to detect the trends underlying the myriad contradictory messages from the plurality of NHS power structures; to accept that policy implementation is a less than rational process deflected by the inevitable exercise of bureaucratic and professional power; to predict the next stage in the political game; and to decide what should be done given their own interests and objectives?

The structure of the book is designed to fulfil several objectives and satisfy a number of audiences. It aims, first, to apply a given theoretical position to what in aggregate amounts to the full range of NHS power arenas, be these functionally, professionally or organisationally defined; and to demonstrate how and why power works, or does not work, therein in particular ways. *In toto* the effect is a matrix of perspectives on the NHS power structures. In this respect the book is intended to be of interest to students of political science and public and social policy. Second and more practically, the objective is that the analysis should provide original insights into the operation of power in the Health Service which would be of use to politicians, bureaucrats, managers and professionals as they engage with this most politicised of welfare institutions or study it from the safe haven of a course in higher education. Finally there is the general informed reader who, while they may suffer some disillusionment when faced with the permanent and inescapable political problem which this book argues besets the NHS, would nonetheless gain a realistic understanding of what may lie behind the latest twist in the NHS saga.

A number of individuals have given generously of their time to comment on drafts of chapters and reorientate the higher flights of analytical fancy that some contained. Most particularly, I would like to thank Ken Hesketh, John Spence, Glenn Douglas, Neil Snee, David Thompson and Ian Young of Medway NHS Trust. Others who have contributed to my continuing NHS education are William Bird, John Bragg, Mark Outhwaite, Barry Page, Sir William Staveley and Glen Stone. Jeremy Kendall helped me to see how economists see things in the NHS. For the rigours of compiling the shifting sands of the references my thanks go to Paula Loader and Barbara Holland and for advice on statistical sources to Barbara Wall. Lastly, this book owes much to the help of my wife Charlotte, who not only carried out much of the grindingly tedious library work and indexing, but also maintained a cheerful irreverence towards the serious academic.

The book draws upon work that I have published elsewhere and, in particular, the articles: 'The politics of purchasing in the National Health Service', *Policy and Politics*, **21**(3): 171–84 (Chapter 2); 'Medicine and the state: redefining the concordat', *Public Policy and Administration*, **10**(3): 60–87 (Chapter 5); "The politics of community care: social rights and welfare limits', *Policy and Politics*, **22**(2): 119–31 (Chapter 7); 'The private sector and the NHS: redefining the welfare state', *Policy and Politics*, **23**(1): 17–30 (Chapter 8).

1

The Politics of Change in the Health Service

Introduction

Change is a seemingly permanent feature of NHS life. Organisations are revamped, funding flows redirected and lines of accountability redrawn as the political tide sweeps remorselessly backwards and forewords. Acronyms appear and disappear overnight as the fraught politics of the NHS demand that a new working group be established or a redundant committee be dispatched. Media interest is constant and for Health Ministers and their senior officials more than any others, inactivity is not an option. If the never-ending public clamour for improved state health services is to be assuaged, policies must be produced, lobbies satisfied and still further promises made.

Yet beneath this frenetic activity lies a system of power relations which change but little as they act to interpret and direct the surface politics of the Health Service. As the cardboard cities of policy are hastily erected, it is these power relations that determine which shaky structures will be given the scaffolding to survive and which will be crumpled, trampled and forgotten. Combining the theatre of illusion with the dramatic substance of genuine power, the NHS is an intensely politicised institution.

The purpose of this book is to explain how the politics of change in that institution works. What is the logic governing the ebb and flow of the underlying forces? How do they interact to promote one policy but to subvert another? What is the relationship between the good intentions of the legislators and the reality of power in the NHS?

In addressing these questions, this chapter opens with the 1988 Review of the NHS, the publication of the White Paper *Working for Patients* and the events leading up to the 1990 NHS and Community Care Act. Here was the legislation which has initiated a period of unprecedented organisational change in the Health Service. Second, the chapter introduces this book's analysis of the fundamental political problem which besets both the welfare state and the NHS. Third, it examines the implications of that analysis for the Health Service, the position of the NHS's major power groups within it, and the pressures for a fresh solution to the problem which led ultimately to the 1990 Act.

Review and reform

When Margaret Thatcher announced the Review of the NHS in January 1988, she was not launching it into entirely uncharted waters. The Health Service had experienced organisational reform before: first in 1974 and then again in 1982. Following the 1974 reorganisation, the Regional Hospital Boards and the Boards of Governors of Teaching Hospitals were brought under the single authority of the Regional Health Authorities (RHAs); the functions of the executive councils were taken over by the Family Practitioner Committees; and 90 Area Health Authorities (AHAs) were created with boundaries that paralleled those of the Local Authorities. Then in 1982 the AHAs were removed and replaced by 192 District Health Authorities (DHAs) (Figure 1.1).

But the Review had ambitions which took it considerably beyond the realm of organisational structures. In a sense it had no choice. From the mid-1980s there had developed a strong body of public and official opinion which saw the NHS as underfunded and ill-equipped to meet the legitimate expectations of its consumers. The frequent reiteration in the House of Commons by Margaret Thatcher and her ministers that there had been a continuing real increase in the NHS budget cut little ice. Against this could be set, for example, the view of the House of Commons Social Services Committee that between 1981–82 and 1987–88 the hospital and community health services in England had been underfunded by £1.896 billion (Social Services Committee of the House of Commons, 1988). By late 1987 the Government was confronted by a clearly disaffected medical profession and was constantly besieged by media reports of hospital inadequacies. The gap between the demand for health care and the available supply was reaching the limit of its political tolerance.

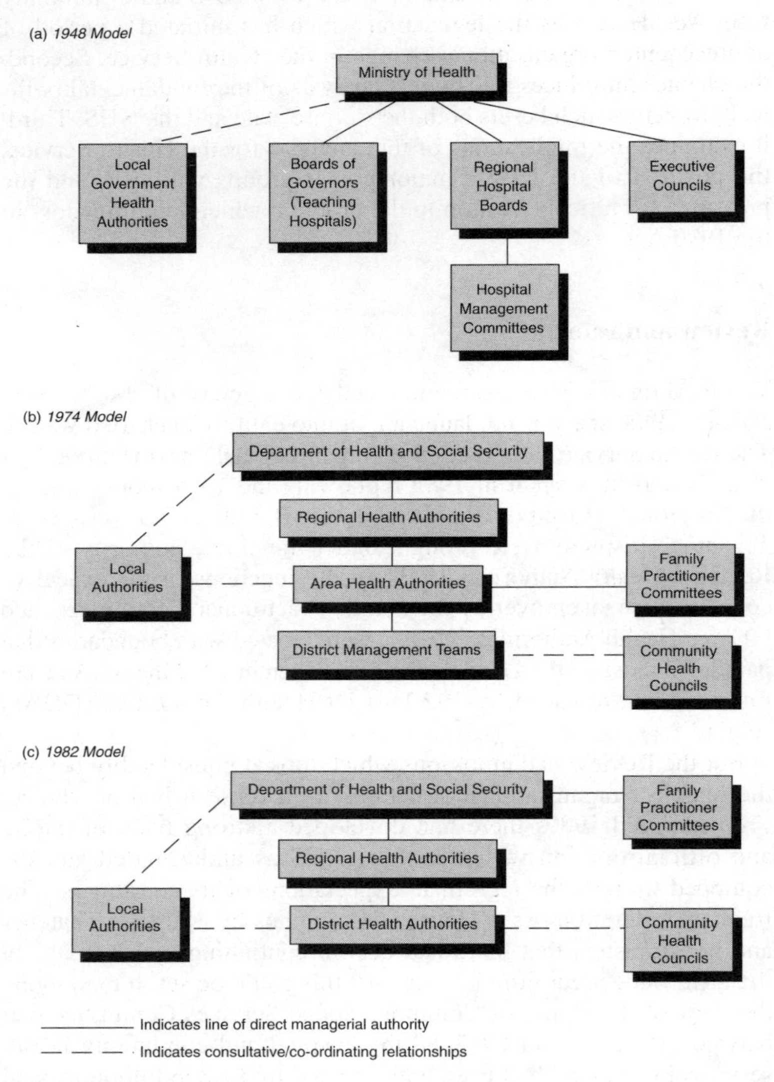

Source: Klein 1989, 84.

Figure 1.1 The changing structure of the National Health Service (England) 1948–1991

In addressing this problem the Review had a choice: it could focus on the demand side, on the supply side or on both. Initially, at least, Mrs Thatcher set no limit on its brief and readily included the funding base of the NHS within its brief. This was to be expected given the influence of the New Right intellectuals of the Conservative Party who, since the mid-1980s, had argued that the mechanisms of the market could be injected equally well into the provision of health care as into other areas of social policy (see for example Elwell, 1986; Green, 1986, 1988; Goldsmith and Willetts, 1988; Letwin and Redwood, 1988). Their critique suggested that in the NHS bureaucratic inertia and professional dominance had produced a service unresponsive to the needs of the consumer. What was required, they maintained, was a devolution of money and power to the consumer, greater patient choice of health care provider, and a corresponding diminution of the power of both doctors and managers as competition becomes a reality. As in all markets, the reconciliation of demand and supply was to be achieved through the price mechanism: individual consumers would limit or increase the demand they placed upon the Health Service in the light of the price of the available supply.

Clearly the New Right position and the NHS ethic of health care free at the point of delivery have quite different conceptions of how the balance between demand and supply is to be struck. On the one hand, the New Right assumes that the individual self-regulates his/her demand; on the other, the NHS right to health care assumes that self-regulation is not required because it is the duty of the state to generate the appropriate supply. For the self-regulation of demand to work, the financial structure of health care has to ensure that an individual's choice produces a cost to that individual. While the NHS is funded out of general taxation no such link can exist and it was therefore an essential prerequisite of the implementation of the New Right ideas that the method of funding the NHS should be reviewed.

In this context, the change of direction by the Review and its subsequent focus on organisation rather than finance graphically illustrates the difficulties faced by the state should it attempt to redefine publicly its responsibilities for health care (Butler, 1992: 8–9). The political costs of such a move, without appropriate ideological preparation of the public, are bound to be prohibitively high. When *Working for Patients* was published in 1989, therefore, the diagnosis of the problem of excess demand remained but the recommended treatment, though radical in organisational terms, did not challenge the traditional view of the state's duty to the financing of health care. The White Paper observed that despite the expansion of the NHS 'it has become increasingly clear that more needs to be done because of rising demand and an ever-widening range of treatments made possible by advances in medical technology. It has also been recognised that simply injecting more and more money is not, by itself, the answer' (Department of Health [DoH], 1989a: 2). Instead, it concludes, 'it is clear that the *organisation of the NHS – the way it delivers health care* to the individual patient – also needs to be reformed' (*ibid.*: 3, emphasis added). One must infer from this that the solution offered is one where the rising demand will be dealt with through a more efficient organisation of the available supply.

Two guiding themes run through the various *Working for Patients* policy documents detailing the reforms which are to be implemented. First, and initially low key, there is the idea of the internal market of the NHS advocated by Enthoven with its attendant notions of organisational independence, competition and consumer power which acted as a powerful influence on the direction taken by the Review (Enthoven, 1985). Second, there is the introduction of more efficient management systems in terms of (a) devolved operational management and (b) 'for the first time a clear and effective chain of management command running from Districts through Regions to the Chief Executive and from there to the Secretary of State' (*ibid.*: 13). Although the two themes are generally presented as different but complementary aspects of the same policy, in reality they are redolent of the political compromises within it.

The structural foundation of the reforms and the prerequisite of any kind of market mechanism was the division between the purchaser and provider functions (Figure 1.2a and b). To begin with, the purchasing agencies were the DHAs buying secondary care services, the Family Practitioner Committees (FPCs – soon to become Family Health Service Authorities (FHSAs)) buying primary care services, and the GP Fundholders both buying some secondary care and providing primary care. Each was required to identify the needs of their catchment populations and enter into contracts with health care providers to supply the services to meet those needs. Purchasers were expected to secure the best and most cost-effective services for their patients and this could mean buying services, in the case of DHAs, 'from its own hospitals, from other authorities' hospitals, from self-governing hospitals or from the private sector' (*ibid.*: 33).

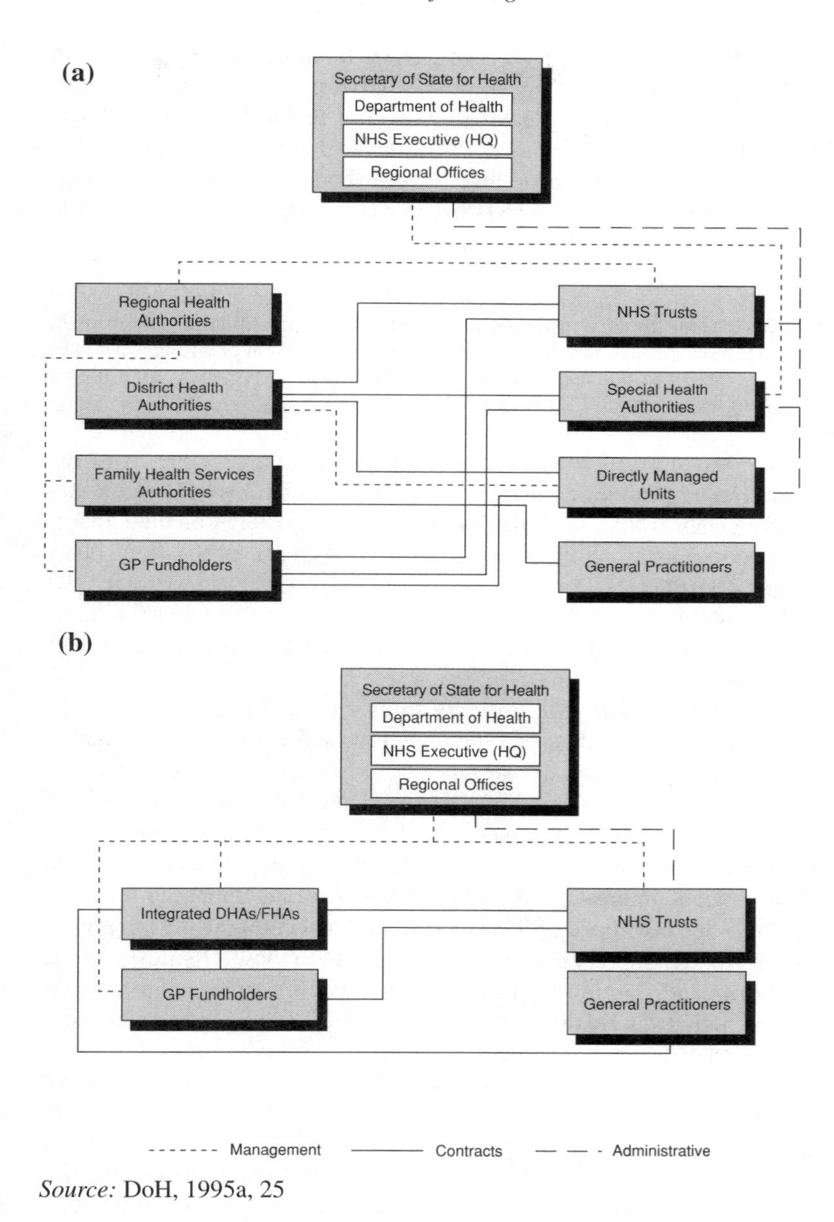

Source: DoH, 1995a, 25

Figure 1.2 Structure of the National Health Service: **(a)** 1991–96, **(b)** 1996 onwards

On the provider side, existing NHS hospital, community, and ambulance units were to become self-governing Trusts with a separate legal identity and greater powers and responsibilities to determine their own future. In the early days of the reforms great play was made of their independence. Hence the National Health Service Management Executive's (NHSME) *NHS Trusts: A Working Guide* issued in 1990 enthusiastically stated that:

> Whilst remaining fully within the NHS, Trusts differ in one fundamental respect from directly managed units – they are operationally independent. Trusts have the power to make their own decisions – right or wrong! – without being subject to bureaucratic procedures, processes or pressures from higher tiers of management. (NHSME, 1990a)

This independence was to be used to generate revenue from the provision of services contracted by purchasers who would be mainly NHS agencies but could also include private patients or their insurance companies, private hospitals, employers and other NHS hospital Trusts.

Meanwhile in the field of primary care, GPs, dentists, opticians and pharmacists who had always been self-employed, independent providers were to continue to be so.

Although *Working for Patients* studiously avoids mentioning the word 'market', it is clear that the organisational units of the purchaser-provider arrangement were designed to promote market-type activities. (Interestingly, this was not just a market 'internal' to the NHS because from the outset both purchasers and providers were encouraged to contract services from the private sector should they deem this to be in their patients' interests.) As part of this new arrangement, all levels of the NHS were stripped of their representational components in order to allow for the more efficient conduct of their new business. Local Authority and Community Health Council (CHC) representatives were dispatched from Health Authorities and FPCs and senior managers were elevated to the new top tier, the Board, of both purchasing agencies (DHAs and FPCs) and providers (Trusts). Boards were to consist of five executive members, five non-executive members (initially selected for the skills they brought to the organisation) and a chairman.

There is no conflict between this market orientation and the second theme's emphasis on greater management efficiency through the devolution of operational control to local organisational units. Where the difficulty emerges is in the balance that is to be struck between the efficient management of the system *as a whole*, publicly funded as it is, and the local management freedoms inherent in any market mechanism. In a prescient article on the 1989 Review, Maynard highlighted the tensions within its recommendations:

> For the market to work it should be untrammelled by regulations that hold down costs and protect particular agencies, for example the London teaching hospitals. But for costs to be contained, cash limits met and public funding maintained, it will be necessary to regulate the market. (Maynard, 1989)

As a taxation-based economic system, therefore, the NHS will always to an extent have to be managed in a top-down manner (disregarding for the moment the numerous political pressures for so doing) and the reforms were always going to be characterised by an uneasy balance between controls and freedoms.

The political problem: citizenship, rights and welfare limits

This, then, was the organisational solution to the perceived difficulties of the NHS in the late 1980s from which so much has flowed in the 1990s. But what exactly was the nature of the political problem which lay behind the Health Service's very visible troubles and what are its implications for the dynamics of change in the Health Service?

The 1990 reorganisation of the NHS was essentially a policy which reconfigured the way in which free health care is delivered to British citizens. Its premise was that the problem of the excess demand for health care can be dealt with through an increase in efficiency achieved by organising the available supply along market principles. Since efficiency-saving exercises must at some stage reach a point where all the surplus fat has been removed, the logic of the policy dictates that this must also be the stage at which the demand for health care either levels out or has a rate of increase conveniently equal to the rate of increase in NHS resources (historically one or two per cent per year). There is no evidence that such a fortuitous and unprecedented coincidence will occur.

The new NHS, like the old one, must therefore fall victim to the dilemma which Klein has expressed in the form of this elegant but simple equation:

> On the one side, are the demands generated both by NHS providers and consumers… . On the other side of the equation, are the financial costs. To the extent that priority is given to satisfying demands, so the financial costs are

> likely to rise. To the extent that the financial commitments are contained, so the political costs of the NHS are likely to rise. (Klein, 1989: 238)

The dilemma is unavoidable because it forms part of the political problem facing the welfare state as a whole. That problem has four components: the rights intrinsic to British citizenship which generate the demand for state services; the competition between political parties for the creation of new rights (and hence new demand); the finite nature of the state purse; and the hegemony of welfare state values which deny both the existence of the problem and the need for a policy solution.

Citizenship can be defined as a reciprocal relationship between the individual and the state. As a citizen, the individual has rights which the state guarantees to fulfil and duties which he/she must carry out for the state. In his seminal work *Citizenship and Social Class* Marshall makes a distinction between the civil rights necessary for individual freedom, the political rights necessary in order to participate in the exercise of political power, and social rights (Marshall, 1950: 5). For Marshall, social rights are:

> the whole range from the right to a modicum of economic welfare and security to the right to share to the full in the social heritage and to live the life of a civilised being according to the standards prevailing in society. (*ibid.*)

The key difference between civil and political rights, on the one hand, and social rights, on the other, is that realisation of the latter requires an active and interventionist state prepared to give the formal status of citizenship a material foundation. In other words, a qualitative shift has to occur in the relationship between a state and its citizens (Van Steenbergen, 1994: 3). Most discussions of social rights agree, with Marshall, that the means used by the state to meet its obligations to its citizens should be the welfare state. Access to welfare services then becomes part of the practical status of citizenship.

The growth of welfare demand is facilitated by the fact that the concept of social rights is infinitely expandable, always flexible and never exclusive. Marshall's classic definition, for example, allows for a myriad of interpretations. There is not, nor has there ever been, any consensus regarding what one might call the 'core' social rights of British citizenship and hence the core identity of the welfare state. This is in marked contrast to civil and political rights where agreement does exist on the fundamental principles of citizenship. Therefore no social right can *a priori* be regarded as off-limits nor can the social rights domain of British citizenship ever be regarded as complete. As a result, in the half-century since the Beveridge Report based the architecture of the welfare state on the three pillars of health, education and social security, there has been a steady, and *ad hoc*, increase in state-recognised social rights unguided and untested by any overarching view of whether one social right should have priority over another.

The second component of the political problem is the electoral character of the British political system itself. Political parties dependent upon a fully enfranchised electorate will always have a strong pragmatic motivation to offer citizens more social rights within the welfare state, and not less, regardless of any single party's ideological stance. As there is a proliferation of interest groups focusing on particular social rights, and as their political sophistication, handling of the media, and targeting of vulnerable areas of parties' policies (of which there are always some) improves, parties find themselves in an upward spiral of competition for the favours, or at least the non-disapprobation, of these groups. In this context, success becomes the presentation of a policy for adding another group deserving of state support to the welfare list before the other party does. (Nursery education is a recent example of this phenomenon.) The overall effect of party competition is to ensure, as Bellamy remarks, that 'the complexity and pluralism of modern societies leads to unresolvable and infinitely expanding claims of rights' (Bellamy, 1993: 71). Each additional social right recognised by the state establishes a new benchmark of welfare state provision which subsequent lobbies for a particular cause can take as their starting point.

On the other side of the political equation to social rights is the social duty to the payment of taxes. Taxation provides the state with the resources with which to meet its obligations to its citizens. Unfortunately, this supply side of the equation has never been able to keep pace with the increase in demand. As a result, between 1951 and 1991 (a period of rising government expenditure when expressed as a proportion of a growing Gross National Product) the share of total government spending accorded to the welfare state doubled from 28.7 per cent to 58.8 per cent (Table 1.1).

But although the demands on the welfare services constantly outstripped the supply of state resources available, public awareness of the fundamental nature of the problem was restricted by the dominance of welfare state values themselves.

Table 1.1 Government spending on the welfare state as a proportion of public expenditure 1951–91

	1951	*1961*	*1971*	*1981*	*1991*	*1994*
Social security	11.8	15.8	16.4	31.1	32.1	34
Health and personal social services	10.1	9.0	11.5	13.4	13.8	14
Education	6.8	9.8	11.7	14.3	12.9	13
Total	28.7	34.6	39.6	58.8	58.8	61

Source: Allsop, 1995, Table 4.2: 68 and Central Statistical Office, 1996, Table 6. 22: 126

This hegemony assumes that the expansion of social rights, and hence of welfare state spending, is a good in its own right requiring little or no justification. Where there have been debates about the welfare state, as there were in the early 1980s, these have largely centred on the appropriate mechanisms for funding and delivering the service rather than on the principles on which it is founded (see for example Offe, 1983; Mishra, 1984; Johnson, 1987). Essentially the problems of the welfare state were seen as technical and administrative, and in this sense reflected the traditional style in the social policy field (which had most to say on the matter), rather than as raising fundamental political issues about the nature of welfare itself. To gain an alternative perspective which does not take the values of the welfare state as given, and therefore a perspective which accords these values a relative rather than an absolute analytical status, one has to turn instead to historians writing about the ideological conflicts between liberalism and the early proponents of the welfare state (see for example Briggs, 1961: 232–42; Rimlinger, 1971: 56–61).

Elsewhere, the hegemony of the belief in the state's blanket responsibility for social rights has prevented the emergence of a clear political understanding of the problems inherent in the welfare state. Periodic attempts by the New Right to bring different and, they would argue, more fundamental issues on to the agenda and to expand the parameters of the debate (as in the case of the NHS Review) have so far achieved only short term visibility and have achieved noticeably little impact either on the way the debate is conducted in academic or parliamentary circles or on the inexorable growth of welfare spending (see for example Elwell, 1986; Green,

1986, 1988; Letwin and Redwood, 1988; Redwood, 1988; Green *et al.*, 1990; No Turning Back Group, 1990).

In general, then, the political problem facing the welfare state can be summarised as follows (Figure 1.3).

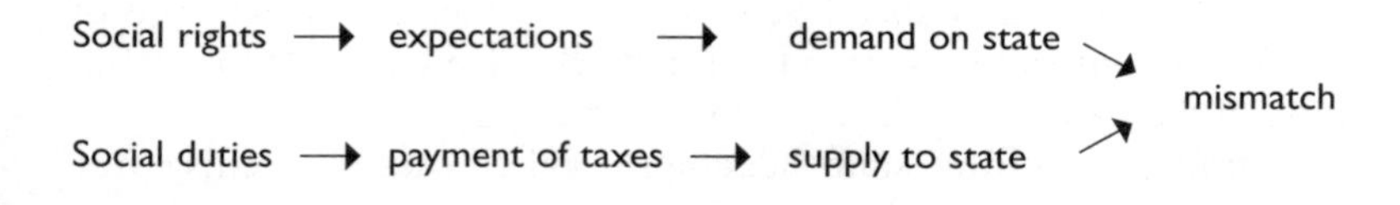

Figure 1.3 The political problem

What are the implications of this analysis for the NHS and what does it tell us about the operation of power therein?

Power and change in the Health Service

As a central part of the welfare state, the Health Service experiences the full effect of the political problem outlined above. In the absence of a government view on how best to manage the gap between health care demand and supply, it has been left to the power structures of the NHS which, by definition, determine its patterns of resource allocation, to evolve their own system solution. Effectively the politicians have, not surprisingly, delegated the political problem.

The operation of the political dynamic for growth in the Health Service takes a familiar form. Neither the National Health Service Act of 1946 nor its successor Act of 1977 actually defines the nature of health, illness and care: what is and what is not the responsibility of the state. Given that in creative hands the range of human conditions and requirements encompassed by these terms can be expanded almost indefinitely, the potential statutory scope of the Health Service, regardless of the demands actually placed upon it, is correspondingly unlimited. Admittedly the 1977 Act did attempt to limit the responsibility of the Secretary of State 'to promote the establishment of a comprehensive health service 'by adding the caveats', to such an extent as he considers necessary to meet all reasonable requirements' and 'such facilities... as he considers are appropriate as part of the health service', but the practical benefit of such powers in the face of the public expectations generated by the NHS and its associated myths are negligible. There is no necessary conflict between the statutory duties of the NHS and that most inclusive of definitions of health by the World Health Organisation, the Alma Ata declaration which states that health consists of a 'state of complete physical, mental and social well being, not merely the absence of disease and infirmity'. Hence the Health Service has no 'core' definition of the citizen's social right to health care.

Within the welfare state hegemony, NHS values promise free comprehensive health care from the cradle to the grave. Whatever is required to achieve that goal is to be supplied by the state at the behest of a beneficent medical profession and the citizen is not only relieved of any responsibility for limiting individual demand but is actively encouraged to register it. The political origins of these values reside in a British model of health care which emphasised the obligation of public authorities to make provision for the community at large, rather than in a model centred on individual rights to health care underpinned by insurance contributions (Klein, 1989: 5–6). Unlike the health care systems of other European countries, the NHS is funded mainly from public taxation rather than from social insurance or from a combination of social insurance, private insurance and taxation. In the ideological arena, this arrangement is used to reinforce the principle that there should be no financial linkage between the individual demand for health care and its supply from the NHS. By removing individual responsibility from the ideological equation, NHS values by definition set no limits on individual demand.

So comprehensive have the social rights and expectations of the Health Service become that they have developed an emotive as well as an intellectual power which can easily be translated into a volatile political issue. Embodied within the NHS values is the promise of, if not mortality, then a mortal life which can be supported and extended in many and various ways. Suffering is outlawed and it is confidently asserted that the Hobbesian notion that life is 'nasty, brutish and short' can be rendered untrue for each and every one of us.

Once established, such values are difficult to oppose within a democratic, multi-party system and, even in the context of the welfare state, must surely be the biggest hostage to fortune in post-war British government; though, admittedly, it is unlikely that Aneurin Bevan was aware of the steamroller dynamic inherent in the policy he fought so tenaciously to get adopted. The assumption in

1948 was that there existed a finite amount of ill-health in the land, that this could be reduced by improved health care and that thereafter the maintenance of the good health of the population would be a relatively simple matter (Thwaites, 1987: 8). Disillusionment soon followed. In 1948–9, the year following the foundation of the NHS, the number of prescriptions tripled and a huge demand for the now free medicines, dentures and spectacles became manifest (Higgins and Ruddle, 1991: 19). Some kind of rationing was then inevitable and the debate of the early 1950s centred around whether charging or queuing was the appropriate mechanism. In the absence of a preparedness to challenge the already powerful values of the Health Service, waiting lists became the preferred option and were consciously adopted as the means for limiting demand (*ibid.*).

The main elements that were to fuel the politics of change in the Health Service were now present: the dynamic of NHS growth was established and the dominating political problem of the demand–supply mismatch was clearly visible. How would the major power groups in the NHS arena respond to these pressures?

There are four power groups in the arena which, in the context of these pressures, interact to create the politics of the Health Service: the politicians, the bureaucrats, the medical profession, and the administrators or managers. Other power groups of course exist but are not central to the politics of the NHS because they cannot directly determine either the demands placed upon the system or the supply of resources to it: to that extent their power is diminished.

The politicians are important because they control the broad parameters of the political game: the contours of the decision-making structures, the formal rules and objectives applied therein, and the total amount of financial resources available in the NHS system. Theoretically, they can also try to influence the ideology of the Health Service although in practice their capacity to do so is much reduced by the prevailing hegemony. It is their responsibility to ensure that the social rights to health care promised by the state are duly delivered and to do so they require some kind of an apparatus of bureaucratic control. This bureaucracy must always include the ability of specific intervention at the local level in order that politicians can be seen to respond to individual social rights issues. Second, those who man the bureaucracy, particularly its middle tiers, have the power to influence the general pattern of the allocation of resources within the system and the interpretation of its rules and objectives. Like the politicians, the bureaucrats deal primarily with the supply side of the political equation.

Not so the medical profession. Through their clinical decisions, doctors define both the demand that is placed upon the Health Service and the detailed disposal of resources. It is the GPs and the consultants who, on a day-to-day basis, provide a practical interpretation of the citizen's social right to health care. This is an ultimate system power which the state recognised and incorporated into the structure of the NHS at its foundation. In so doing, the state was bowing to the inevitable. Having accepted responsibility for the social right to health care and raised its citizens' expectations, it was then dependent on the medical profession to control the situation: not a very strong negotiating position. The political consequence was, as Klein observes, that 'implicit in the structure of the NHS' was the bargain between the state and the medical profession which ensured that 'while central government controlled the budget, doctors controlled what happened within that budget' (Klein, 1989: 82). There was no assumption on the part of the medical profession, however, that it was the public duty of doctors to make certain that resource supply and citizen demand matched. They would help to establish a rough and ready relationship between the two but the responsibility for the solution to the political equation remained that of the state.

As the demand for health care has progressively outstripped the NHS supply, the state has sought alternative ways of balancing the equation. One alternative has been to try and persuade doctors themselves to work within fixed budgets, the other has been to use a relatively new power group, the managers, to insist that doctors do so. Neither option has been successful but the introduction of general management in the early 1980s formally established managers as a power group in the political arena of the Health Service. They replaced the traditional NHS administrators who had tacitly accepted the lead role of the medical profession in the business of resource allocation. Managers do not accept that doctors should have that role and their attempt to limit the autonomy of the medical profession is now central to the politics of change in the NHS.

However, for two decades following the foundation of the NHS the relationship between the four power groups was amicable enough as they combined to manage the demand–supply mismatch. The medical profession used the authority of clinical judgement to dampen demand to an acceptable level, the administrators facilitated the doctors' work, the bureaucrats weaved their planning web around the positions of medical interest, and the politicians danced their dance in the embrace of party consensus. Then gradually the logic of the dynamic of welfare growth began to have its impact. By the early 1970s the medical profession was aware that its ability to manage the widening gap between the public's ever increasing expectations of the NHS and the not-so-rapidly expanding supply of health care was coming under severe strain. In its 1970 report on NHS financing the British Medical Association (BMA) noted that 'the NHS has never since its early years been able to fully cope with the rising demands that it, and the parallel development of new methods of treatment, were responsible for stimulating' (British Medical Association, 1970, section 6.1). Other observers noted the growing dilemma over rationing in the NHS (Maxwell, 1974; Cooper, 1975). Then, in an unprecedented and perhaps unwise move into this sensitive area, the politicians decided to take to the floor.

In 1976 they gave formal public recognition to the issue with the publication of *Priorities for the Health and Personal Social Services in England: a Consultative Document* in which Barbara Castle, then Secretary of State for Health and Social Services, explicitly acknowledged that 'demand will always outstrip our capacity to meet it' (Department of Health and Social Services [DHSS], 1976: iii). The document proudly proclaimed that 'it was a new departure', that it was 'the first time an attempt had been made to establish rational and systematic priorities throughout the health and personal social services' (*ibid.*: section 1). Indeed it was, and in that respect was a political step into the unknown. But what it failed to recognise or discuss, and here showed an impressive naivety, was the enormous gap between the proclamation, on the one hand, and the enforcement and legitimation of priorities, on the other. Priority setting is, after all, rationing by any other name in that is a statement about the selective allocation of scarce resources in a situation of excess demand over supply. It is, consequently, a direct affront to the principle enshrined in the NHS values that there should be unrestricted access to health care. Furthermore, it is a public and visible affront in contrast to the covert and disguised approach of the traditional rationing method. Not surprisingly, therefore, the politicians backed off the floor, at one and the same time demonstrating both the difficulties of publicly confronting the basic political problem of the NHS and their lack of power to deal with it. Following the 1979 election and the end of party consensus on the NHS, they have never reappeared despite recent requests for a return performance on rationing.

In the early and mid-1980s, while the medical profession continued its invisible task of demand control, a combination of bureaucrats and the emerging class of managers were given the job of making more efficient use of the existing supply of resources though a range of managerial initiatives. These included the annual review process, performance indicators, 'efficiency savings', restrictions on doctors' prescribing rights, compulsory competitive tendering for hospital support services and cost improvement programmes (Harrison, 1988: Ch. 4). The impact of such measures on the demand–supply mismatch, however, was always going to be short-lived because, as Thwaites observes, 'each step forward in efficiency is frustrated by two steps backwards in the face of the onrush of expectation' (Thwaites, 1987: 19).

Perhaps greater weight could have been attached, at least initially, to the recommendations of the inquiry into the management of the NHS, chaired by Sir Roy Griffiths, which reported in 1983. As well as ushering in the new general managers, Griffiths roundly lectured doctors on their responsibilities. Prior to his report the so-called 'Cogwheel' system introduced in the 1960s for giving doctors information about the effects of their decisions, and the consensus management team approach that formed part of the 1974 reorganisation of the NHS had attempted to persuade doctors into management in diplomatic fashion. Now Griffiths insisted:

> Greater involvement of doctors is… critical to effective management at local level… . Their decisions largely dictate the use of all resources… . They must accept the management responsibility which goes with clinical freedom. This implies active involvement in securing the most effective use and management of all resources. (DHSS, 1983a: 18–19)

In stating categorically that an explicit link should be forged between clinical decisions, which determine the expressed demand for health care, and the financial resources available, Griffiths was asking for a radical reshaping of the doctor's political role. Covert demand control is one thing, but public rationing quite another. But as there was no incentive attached to such a new role, and fairly obvious disincentives, the medical profession's reaction to the Griffiths proposals was, certainly in the short term, lukewarm.

By the end of the 1980s, two things are clear. First, that despite the continuing real increase in NHS expenditure (Table 1.2.), it was not keeping pace with people's expectations.

Table 1.2 Percentage change of 'real' NHS cost in 10-year period, 1953–93

	Total NHS (%)	*NHS per person (%)*
1953–63	46	38
1963–73	60	52
1973–83	51	51
1983–93	37	33

Source: Office of Health Economics, 1995, Box 7.

Second, that the traditional alliance for dealing with the health care demand–supply mismatch could no longer cope with the situation and had broken down. Politicians, bureaucrats, doctors and managers now co-existed in a state of simmering tension. Politically, something had to be done.

Conclusions

The chosen route was the 1989 Review of the NHS and the remainder of this book will explore the effect of the Review and the subsequent legislation on the politics of change in the Health Service. That legislation established a new organisational framework for the Health Service based on the division between purchaser and provider, devolved operational management, and a continuing drive towards greater efficiency. But what it did not do was to address the fundamental political problem of the NHS.

This chapter has set out the main components of that problem and the analysis which will be used to understand how it impacts on the different NHS arenas. Driving that analysis is the dynamic for growth in the welfare state. Firmly ensconced in the British concept of citizenship is a view of social rights which, through its vagueness, its infinite mutability and its dominance, fuels a continually rising demand on the vehicle for its realisation: the welfare state. Established now for 50 years, the welfare state is as much an ideological force as it is an institution and contributes mightily to the escalation of the demand. As each new right is added to the welfare list, so a new threshold of orthodoxy is established below which the political parties, sensitive to the needs of their electorate, are anxious not to fall. Indeed, the search for new rights has become an area of intense party competition.

If the supply of tax revenues were infinite this would not be a problem. But it is the mismatch between the demand for welfare and the supply of state resources which, with the electorally acceptable ceiling of taxation highly visible, now exercises all the political parties. The experience of the Health Service is a quintessential example of this fundamental political problem.

Like the rest of the welfare state, the NHS has no defined core of healthcare social rights for which it is responsible. Given the impetus for the growth of these rights, fostered and legitimised by the hegemony of welfare, the Health Service is obliged continually to extend the menu of physical and mental conditions for which it takes responsibility. As the expectations and demands of citizens has risen, so the original system of power relations within the NHS has found it increasingly difficult to manage the political problem of the demand–supply mismatch.

Often fevered party competition for the mantle of NHS protector ('the NHS is safe in our hands' and so on), coupled with the unchallenged status of NHS values, has meant that politicians are unable to scrutinise and form policy on the demand side of the equation because to do so would mean questioning the social rights on which the demand is based. Doctors, meanwhile, have found the escalating demand difficult to deal with and the essence of their power, their clinical authority, less effective than in days of yore. Unlike doctors, neither bureaucrats nor managers can directly control demand but they do have the power to structure the supply of health care resources in an attempt to ration what is available. Inevitable tensions have then arisen between the demand identified by the doctors' clinical judgement and the resources allocated by the bureaucrats and managers.

Disconsolate they may have been but at least, it could be argued, the principal actors in the NHS drama were performing on a familiar organisational stage which, although it had undergone some scene-shifting over the years, was still recognisably that of the 1948 NHS. With the 1990 NHS and Community Care Act that stage was abruptly removed. Not only was the new one quite different but its props and furniture appeared to change with alarming rapidity. What is the organisational logic at work in the post-1990 situation and how does it impact on the power structures of the Health Service?

2

Purchasing

Introduction

The decision to introduce an internal market based on the division between the purchaser and provider of health care brought into sharp focus the key political problem of the NHS: that the demand for health care will always exceed the supply, that a rationing mechanism is therefore required to resolve the difference between the two, but that the explicit rationing of resources is unacceptable to the health care rights embodied in the concept of British citizenship. In the past the resolution of this conundrum was achieved covertly: rationing took place, but it was in no-one's interest to advertise the fact. What the reforms have achieved is the creation of a role, that of the purchasing agent, which takes clear and unequivocal responsibility for the allocation of resources, which must, given excess demand, make overt choices about the rationing of scarce resources and which will, inevitably, conflict with the universalistic values of the welfare state.

A new political game of resource allocation has been initiated where the rules remain unclear, the range of potential participants is vast, and where there exists no set of values to guide and legitimise the development and application of purchasing procedures. For the first time in the history of the NHS, a policy has been introduced which directly addresses the issue of the control of the demand for health care apparently unaware of the challenge this presents to the hegemonic order of the welfare state. The result is uncertainty, confusion and an inability satisfactorily to confront the rationing choices which purchasers have to make.

The purpose of this chapter is to analyse the contribution of purchasing to the politics of change in the Health Service: first, by identifying the main components of the new political game of purchasing and the inconsistencies and compromises therein; second, by examining the political difficulties inherent in explicit rationing in the present political culture and the consequent implications for the power structure of the NHS. Has purchasing rent the veil of medical power asunder or has the challenge been blunted by the historic inertia of the Health Service?

The context

Decisions about the allocation and, given excess demand, the rationing of health care resources in the Health Service occur at five levels (Figure 2.1).

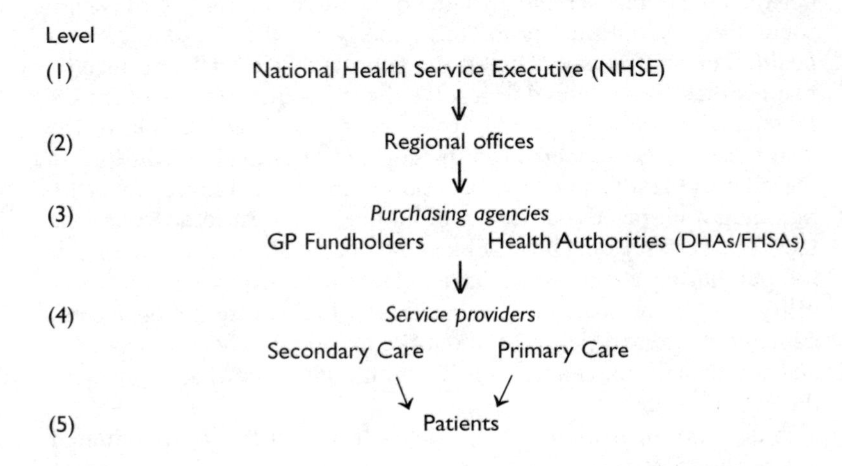

Figure 2.1 Levels of rationing

At the national level, the annual amount available to the NHS is the result of competition between the various government departments and the priority accorded to the Department of Health (DoH). On average, the annual growth rate in real public health expenditure since 1949 has been 3.5 per cent (Whynes, 1992). Up to 1976, the regional distribution of NHS funds followed historical patterns.

Thereafter until 1990, allocations to Regional Health Authorities (RHAs) were based on the formula produced by the Resource Allocation Working Party (RAWP) which progressively changed the balance of funding between regions. In 1990, following a review conducted in 1988 (Coopers and Lybrand, 1988), the formula was revised and further adjustments between regions followed.

While there is a common formula for the rationing of resources to the regional tier, there is no common approach to guide the subsequent allocations by regions to the purchasing agencies. The newly formed Health Authorities have inherited two quite different methods for the funding of their District Health Authority (DHA) and Family Health Service Authority (FHSA) components. DHA funding is progressively being allocated on the basis of some form of weighted capitation (a population-based formula incorporating statistical proxies for health care needs) but the precise formula differs from region to region. In the case of FHSAs, allocations are made on the basis of historical levels of expressed demand which will have varied for numerous reasons. Although some attempt has been made to demonstrate a statistical relationship between certain FHSA characteristics and level of funding (Judge and Benzeval, 1991), this is unconvincing and perhaps best viewed as an exercise in *post hoc* rationalisation through the codification of past allocation decisions (Sheldon and Carr-Hill, 1991a: 25). In the case of GP Fundholders, the parallel use of historical levels of activity and referrals to establish funding levels has produced variations between practices such that the largest budget per patient was more than 1.5 times as high as the smallest (Glennerster *et al.*, 1992: 22). In short, the rationing of resources to purchasing agencies is a highly variable and locally determined process.

At the fourth level, the purchasing agencies of secondary care have to decide how they are going to distribute their funds between the services available and, in certain cases, whether some services will be funded at all. In primary care there is less discretion available to the Health Authority purchaser given the detailed constraints of the national GP Contract which the Health Authority administers. It is left to general practitioners to structure the supply of primary care through their discretionary take-up of the numerous fees for item-of-services available within the Contract.

The final and most critical part of this cascade of rationing is that of the patient his/herself. While all of the levels have a rationing issue to address, it is at the level of the individual patient that the collision between rights and resources has been most sensitive.

Traditionally, the medical profession accepted the responsibility for handling that collision. Its methods were informal and non-bureaucratic, largely disguised and legitimised the rationing activity under the cloak of clinical judgement, and protected the rationing levels above the individual patient from excessive public scrutiny. It is instructive to explore how this mechanism for dealing with the demand–supply mismatch worked, and works, as a context for the subsequent discussion of the problems faced by purchasing agencies.

The first point for the expression of most health care demand are the GPs who act as gatekeepers both for their own service and, by referral, for those of the hospital consultants. The consultants, in turn, then act as further gatekeepers either to their own service or to that of another consultant. Where, as in most cases, the service is not immediately available, the patient is placed on a waiting list which thus becomes the physical manifestation of the demand–supply mismatch. In theory, this method of dealing with health care demand is the result of impartial clinical decisions unsullied by other factors. In practice, research suggests that access to the supply of health care is determined by a multiplicity of factors such as debarring rules, the personal predilection of the doctor, acceptance of only those cases deemed likely to benefit from particular services, priority classes of need, and knowledge or ignorance of the services available (Rees, 1972: 38–42). The well-documented variations in medical practice, patterns of referral, and use of common surgical procedures are the natural consequence of the social nature of the gatekeeping function and the variety of non-medical criteria employed (McPherson *et al.*, 1981; Andersen and Mooney, 1990).

For political purposes, however, this does not matter, provided that the public continues to believe that such rationing decisions are made on the basis of freely exercised clinical judgement and hence that any restrictions on its access to health care are authoritative and legitimate. Such is the esteem in which medicine is held: it is the only profession whose values have been sufficiently politically robust to control the popular expectations of the NHS.

The new political game

The first chapter has already dealt with the reasons why the 'hidden hand' of medical rationing has become less effective in the last ten years. The upward spiral of citizens' health care rights and expectations has been encouraged by a state bent on proving through The Patient's Charter and The Health of the Nation initiatives that its mission is to care ever more assiduously for the nation's welfare. Hence the NHSE's *Priorities and Planning* 1996–97 guidance, for example, expansively claimed that:

> The purpose of the NHS is to secure, through the resources available, the greatest possible improvement to the physical and mental health of the people of England by promoting health, preventing ill health, diagnosing and treating disease and injury, and caring for those with long term illness and disability: a service to all on the basis of clinical need, regardless of the ability to pay. (NHSE, 1995c: 2)

At the same time there are strong indications that citizens activate their health care rights more frequently because, as a chairman of the British Medical Association (BMA) has pointed out, 'public tolerance of personal suffering is probably at an all time low' (Macara, 1994: 849). A striking example of this phenomenon is the doubling of GPs' night calls from 936 000 in 1989–90 to 1 830 000 in 1993–94 (White, 1995: 22). As the gap between the demand for health care and the available supply has widened, so the ability of the medical profession to carry out its rationing function has come under increasing stress and so the level of public satisfaction with the NHS has declined. Hence we have the apparent 'irreconcilability between the unrelenting flow of complaint that the NHS is being cut and the inexorable increase in government allocations in real terms' (Thwaites, 1987: 11).

Into this politically charged arena has been thrust the new role of the purchasing agency. DHAs, FHSAs and GP Fundholders were given the radical agenda of changing the NHS from a provider-driven to a purchaser-led system. No longer would money be passively allocated in response to further increases in the historical pattern of service delivery. Instead, purchasers were consciously to use a range of new, non-medical skills to identify the needs of the population and to structure the supply of health care to meet those needs. Purchasers, it seemed, would be the dominant players in the political game of the internal market because they would have the financial muscle to make things happen. Providers would no longer passively follow the decisions of their clinicians but would be obliged to tailor their activities to the requirements of their purchasing agencies. What was not addressed was how purchasing agencies would deal with the unprecedented shift from implicit to explicit rationing and the new political agenda thus created. How would they integrate into their operation a task with which the doctors, the most powerful group in the Health Service, were already struggling?

In analysing the way in which purchasing has evolved the discussion will deal, first, with issues of organisation and, second, with the politics behind the various techniques of explicit rationing vying for position and influence.

Organisation

The internal market began with three purchasing agencies in situ: the DHAs, the FHSAs and the GP Fundholders. In exploring the organisational logic, or its absence, in purchasing it is reasonable to ask who was purchasing what on behalf of whom according to what criteria and with what resources. In other words, were the game players operating with a shared logic of type of health care purchased, catchment population, needs assessment, and funding formula? Clearly not. It is not the differences themselves that are important but the absence of rules explaining the nature of the differences.

GP Fundholders were able to purchase for their patients a stipulated list of elective acute service care, generally the more common procedures. Districts, on the other hand, were obliged to purchase the full range of elective care for patients registered with non-fundholding practices as well as all emergency and long-term health care for the whole of their resident populations. FHSAs were to purchase primary care services. So far so good. Although the pieces of the jigsaw did not fit exactly, they were at least part of the same design.

We have already seen how there is no shared logic in the regional distribution of funds to purchasing agencies and hence no symmetry in their capacity to buy services. Similarly, there was, and is, no agreement among purchasers regarding the way in which needs assessments should be undertaken to determine the volume and type of service purchased, bearing in mind that such assessment was a fundamental principle of the reforms. Of the three agencies, only DHAs undertook any kind of formal assessment of the needs of their catchment populations as a prior step to the negotiation of contracts with providers. This is because only Districts had a tradition of this activity (through their Public Health Departments) and therefore the expertise required, and only Districts had received detailed advice on how to do it (see for example NHSME, 1991b, c, d). Setting aside for one moment the fact that different Districts used quite different forms of needs assessment, FHSAs and GP Fundholders in contrast made their purchasing decisions on the basis of historical patterns of demand combined with efficiency considerations rather than needs assessment. So the criteria informing the purchasing decision was quite different depending on the agency. This illogicality was most acute where agencies were purchasing the same type of service – as was the case in the buying of elective care by DHAs and GP Fundholders.

The FHSA's role as a purchaser of primary care was also constrained both by its relative youth as a management agency and by its lack of direct financial power over the independent general practitioner. It was only in 1985 that Family Practitioner Committees (FPCs), as they then were, were given independent status and an explicit brief for managing services and in this respect their performance over the next few years was distinctly patchy (see National Audit Office, 1988). General management was introduced into FPCs in 1989 and the following year they were redesignated FHSAs with their line of accountability now running through the RHAs rather than direct to the Department as had previously been the case. But despite this change in nomenclature, they remained very much the local administrators of a nationally agreed contract between the DoH and GPs, with little direct management control over the services delivered and resources consumed (Audit Commission, 1993), and no management control over the allocation of GPs (Butland, 1993). In the light of this, the development of the FHSA purchaser role was always going to be a difficult area.

A final organisational problem peculiar to the DHAs lay in the critical area of the control of demand. The logic of the internal market dictated that purchasers defined the demand for health care by buying particular types and volumes of activity (supply) from the providers. For this mechanism to work, patients had to follow the purchasers' money. It would not work efficiently if, in the words of the political slogan, 'money followed the patients' since this would generate an alternative and conflicting demand. Yet this, to an extent, is what happened. Unimpressed by the new purchasing arrangements, and initially only loosely included in DHA decision making, GPs would sometimes exercise their power of referral by sending their patients to hospital providers with which their DHA did not have a contract, thus creating what was called an Extra-Contractual Referral (ECR). In effect ECRs made the point that consumer (patient) demand is different from customer (purchaser) demand.

The problem for DHAs was how to bring the two types of demand into line and to do this they needed the cooperation of the GPs. Without that cooperation their chances of achieving any kind of rationing was negligible: the regular overspending on their ECR budgets was in this respect a consistent reminder of their vulnerability to GP power (see for example, Salter, 1991b, 1992a; Auplish and Shires, 1994).

The NHSME's initial response to these flaws in the organisation of purchasing was to advocate mergers, 'healthy alliances' and an enhanced role for regions. Informal mergers between DHAs and FHSAs began almost as soon as the internal market was in place and received formal backing as a policy option early in 1991 from two NHSME documents, *FHSAs: Today's and Tomorrow's Priorities* and *Integrating Primary and Secondary Health Care*, the former offering four possible models of how merger could be organised (Foster, 1991; NHSME, 1991e). Both documents also promoted the rather more ephemeral idea of 'healthy alliances' between all three purchasing agencies, though the possible *modus operandi* remained vague and little more than mutual goodwill. The third option was for RHAs to use their corporate contracts with DHAs and FHSAs to ensure the use of common purchasing criteria, though this still left GP Fundholders outside the magic circle since they did not form part of the corporate planning system (Foster, 1991: 16). In common with other proposals that they should help 'manage the market', RHAs varied in the extent to which they attempted to deal with these issues (Ham and Heginbotham, 1991b: 13–14) and in any case were soon overtaken, or rather eliminated, by the course of events.

The Structure, Functions and Manpower Review of the NHS in 1993 (the 'Langlands Review'), and the legislation which implemented its recommendations in 1996, did not directly address the fundamental organisational problems of purchasing. Admittedly DHAs and FHSAs were merged to form the new unitary Health Authorities but there was no suggestion that their different and incompatible funding mechanisms should be replaced by a common system. Rather the official view was that GP Fundholders should become the dominant force in the purchasing of secondary care because 'the experience of the last four years has shown that purchasing delivers more appropriate services for patients when GPs are involved, and particularly when they are involved by taking on the direct control of resources used by their patients' (NHSE, 1994d: 2). This view left Health Authorities with a residual purchasing role and with a 'need to shift the balance of their activity towards these strategic, monitoring and support [of GPs] roles' (NHSE, 1994e: 2). Health Authorities would remain responsible for local health strategies and were to ensure that all GPs contributed towards these strategies (*ibid.*). Precisely how they were to do this remained unclear since the Fundholders' line of accountability was still to the regional tier. This, meanwhile, had experienced the abolition of RHA's and their replacement with eight regional offices of the NHSE which would oversee through separate 'arms' both purchaser and provider activities. Given that this reform was accompanied by a substantial reduction in regional manpower, and given the continued independence of Fundholders from the general management web of the corporate contract system, it was always unlikely to lead to the imposition of more coherence on purchasers' organisational differences through a strong regional 'management of the market' function.

Techniques of explicit rationing

In the first year of the reforms, most official attention, advice and concern concentrated on providers, with purchasers largely left to their own devices. Once the realisation dawned that the purchasing of health care was an entirely new function for the NHS, a flurry of documents resulted which dealt almost exclusively with DHAs. The reasons for this are not hard to find. Of the three purchasing agencies, Districts had the largest aggregate budget and the greatest visibility through their designated 'champions of the people' role (see for example DoH, 1990a: 4). Furthermore, and crucially, they were publicly and technically new gatekeepers to health care – unlike the other two agencies which relied on the traditional gatekeeping role of the GP, albeit with some modifications. In the case of the FHSAs, the management role had been superficially enhanced but their space for the discretionary purchasing of primary care remained confined by the new GP Contract. In the case of GP Fundholders, although the purchasing role was new it inevitably built upon their existing gatekeeping experience. Most importantly, both FHSAs (via GPs) and GP Fundholders were able to incorporate the political advantages of covert rationing into their purchasing functions. Not so the DHAs, they were obliged to carry out their new purchasing function in the public realm.

Official advice to Districts on purchasing attempted to represent matters in a purely technical light but succeeded only in highlighting the political difficulties of moving to a system of explicit rationing. In this sense the documentation serves as a useful introduction to the dimensions of the new political game. The political issue for DHAs, and now Health Authorities, was how they decided what volume and type of health care they were to purchase. Other parts of the purchasing process – purchasing plans, service specifications, contracts and monitoring – are essentially administrative activities, complex perhaps but bureaucratically soluble. Who gets what is the political issue.

The dominant rhetoric suggested that, as 'champions of the people', DHAs first identify the needs of their resident populations and then purchase the health care to meet those needs. The first intimation that 'needs assessment' might prove to be a technical and political morass came in *The Role of District Health Authorities – Analysis of Issues* which adopted what can be termed the 'the Uncle Tom Cobley approach' whereby every conceivable factor relevant to the assessment of a population's health care needs is listed but no indication is given as to how the different factors should be related or weighted in order to arrive at a decision (NHSME, 1989a, Annex II). Rarely surpassed in terms of its comprehensiveness in later pronouncements, this paper listed eight groups of factors which should be used to build on the work of Directors of Public Health in the assessment of the local need and demand for health care: the population profile, the health status of the population, utilisation of services, views of users, views of service providers, views of outside agencies, unmet needs, and statutory and other mandatory obligations. This list was then repackaged and presented in the more authoritative NHS Review Working Paper *Developing Districts* the following year (DoH, 1990a: 13–15).

Effectively these two documents announced that open season existed in the needs assessment category of the new political game. There was, and is, no authoritative method for resource allocation decisions by purchasers in the post-1990 NHS. The realisation that what was previously the exclusive territory of the clinicians is now, apparently, as yet unclaimed land has prompted intense competition for control over it between a range of very interested participants. The current players are public health physicians and allied members of the medical profession, health economists, advocates of formula funding (largely statisticians) and philosophers. Each group is seeking to use its professional knowledge and authority to define and dominate some or all of the purchasing agenda (Salter, 1991a, 1993b).

It might be assumed that public health physicians would have won hands down. Following the Acheson Report of 1988 (DHSS, 1988), Departments of Public Health were given a central role in the evaluation and monitoring of DHA policy, their annual reports were given added status and, when the reforms arrived they were frequently regarded as the officers in place to deal with the strange animal of purchasing. They were familiar with identifying health care needs using epidemiological data and given the limitations of other needs-related information could argue that 'for the immediate future there is no alternative but to assess needs in the traditional disease process manner using existing data' (Eskin and Bull, 1991: 17). If in doubt, they could always turn to the 15 health targets of the Faculty of Public Health Medicine, derived from the World Health Organisation's *Targets for Health for All*, as authoritative guidelines for action or to a more democratically determined list of targets 'cascading through the NHS' with the help and monitoring of public health medicine (Catford, 1991: 981). Some public health physicians were convinced that they were indeed the protectors of the populace against over-precipitous attempts led by finance officers and planners to draw up contracts which would modify provision (Stevens and Gabbay, 1991: 22). Public health physicians, they warn, must refashion these contracts otherwise 'there is a grave danger that contracts will end up serving the factional interests of health care purchasers and providers, rather than the health care needs of the population [as defined by us]' (*ibid.*).

Further support for a medical dominance of purchasing has come from the burgeoning knowledge industry of 'evidence-based medicine', official protection for the principle of clinical freedom and central sponsorship for the inclusion of doctors in consultative arrangements. The circular *Improving Clinical Effectiveness* announced that the NHSE wished to see better use made of research-based clinical guidelines in the contracting process and pointed purchasing agencies towards the data provided by Effective Health Care Bulletins, Epidemiological Based Needs Assessments, the Cochrane Database, Health of the Nation Key Area Handbooks, and Population Health Outcome Indicators (NHSE, 1993a; see also NHSE, 1994f). At the same time the NHSE was careful to respect the professional sensitivities of doctors and insisted that any changes in contracts, purchasing specifications, schedules of service and activity levels must secure the support of the clinicians involved 'whose freedom to determine the treatment of individual patients must be preserved' (NHSE, 1993a; see also NHSE, 1993b). Furthermore it was regarded as essential that the advice of GPs be incorporated into the construction of health strategies through a variety of possible methods (NHSE, 1993c).

Exclusive professional self-belief is not a characteristic confined to medicine. Health economists too have their share. They exhibit little doubt about either the nature of the purchasing problem or their ability to deal with it. Alan Maynard has argued that:

> The central problem in the resource allocation debate – which non-economists call rationing, is what criteria should be used to allocate resources among competing patients... to determine which patients will be left to die and which patients will be left in pain and discomfort? (Society for Social Medicine, 1990: 187).

While some might demur at assuming responsibility for such difficult decisions, or at least wish to spread the load, Maynard has no doubts. The answer, he claims unequivocably, is the economic approach to the measurement of social need which 'emerges as efficient, equitable, ethical, and unavoidable' (*ibid.*: 188). Likewise, Donaldson and Mooney emphatically staked a claim for the use of economic evaluation in determining priorities in health care and confidently maintained that 'its widespread use will ensure that, no matter what total needs are, health care resources are used in such a way as to maximise the benefits from them' (Donaldson and Mooney, 1991: 1529).

The objective of health economists is to shift the purchasing agenda away from a focus on needs, which they describe as a 'red herring' (*ibid.*: 1530), to 'marginal met need for resources expended' (that is outcomes, costs and benefits) in order to identify 'those interventions which contribute most to reducing need per pound spent' (Donaldson and Farrar, 1991: 3; see also Ferguson and Ryder, 1991). However, in order to operationalise this framework and so compete effectively in the purchasing arena, health economists require quite different data sets to the epidemiologically orientated information used by public health physicians and medical researchers. Except for scattered examples of the Qualitative Life Years (QALY) approach originally pioneered by Williams (Williams, 1985) such data is not readily available and the knowledge base of the health economists to this extent lacks political conviction.

By way of contrast, the supporters of formula funding have argued that their approach uses the manipulation of readily available bodies of data to determine how resources should be allocated and that 'rational formulae' have the advantage that they are easy to administer. As well as these technical benefits, it is claimed that formulae are politically advantageous because they are 'a planning constraint on the exercise of arbitrary power' (Carr-Hill and Sheldon, 1992: 124), can be made available for scrutiny so that the 'rules of the game' are plain to see, and can ease the political pressure associated with discretionary area-by-area, case-by-case decision-making (Sheldon and Carr-Hill, 1991b: 18). Given the history of formula funding in the Health Service, there is clearly some substance to these claims. We saw earlier how formulae have for two decades dominated the regional funding allocations and although there has been much dispute over the formula appropriate to sub-regional resource allocation this has to be seen as normal intra-professional feuding about statistical detail, not about the principle of formula funding itself (see for example Balarajan, 1990; Sheldon and Carr-Hill, 1991c). Pressure has already been exerted for the historical allocations of FHSAs and Fundholders to be subject to some form of weighted capitation (Glennerster *et al.*, 1992: 23) and in terms of regional-purchaser rationing, formula funding would seem to have a bright future. Its usage will of course always be subject to the demands of political reality and its advocates must realise that they are engaged in a process of political bargaining. Hence the health economists of York University should not have been too surprised (as they seem to have been) when, in 1995, their new and much prized formula for allocations from regions to purchasers was only selectively adopted by the NHSE for reasons of political pragmatism (Appleby, 1995; Hunter, 1995).

Although formulae have not so far been used as a means for rationing purchaser resources to the fourth level of 'service providers' (Figure 2.1), there is no reason why supporters of this approach should not pursue the logic of their position to advocate such a course of action. One obvious way forward would be an alliance between formulae supporters and public health physicians where a codified approach to epidemiological data would be used to produce priority areas for funding. Rather more ambitious would be a British version of the Oregon experiment where an elaborate formula combined consumer views with economic evaluation to produce a hierarchy of health care interventions to guide funding decisions

(McBride, 1990; Dixon and Welch, 1991; Klein, 1991, 1992). It may yet happen in the UK. One suggested framework for the assessment of health care priorities in Scottish Health Boards showed how government priorities, consumer opinion, need and economic appraisal could act as weighted components of what amounted to a priority-setting formula (Breen, 1991).

The role of philosophers in the struggle for control of the purchasing agenda has largely been a subordinate one, reacting to the claims of the other participants and questioning their validity rather than asserting a particular ethical approach (see for example Relman, 1990; Society for Social Medicine, 1990). Unlike the other three groups, they lack both the ability to support their arguments with exhaustively manipulated data, presently a symbol of credibility, and the means to translate them into practical policy statements.

The attempts by the National Health Service Management Executive (NHSME) to act as the arbiter between the warring factions has led to a series of impressively inscrutable statements about the relationship between needs assessment and purchasing, illustrating the difficulties of official pronouncements on explicit rationing (NHSME, 1991b, c, d). Rather than come down on one side or the other, the NHSME retained the basic Uncle Tom Cobley approach but refined it through the use of idiosyncratic definitions and categorisations in order, presumably, to try to convey the impression that order and good sense prevail. So, for example, *Moving Forward: Needs, Services and Contracts* outlined three elements of needs assessment. The first, 'epidemiological assessments', is an indecipherable forced marriage between ideas drawn from public health and health economics in that it is: 'based on the ability to benefit from health care and [reflects] what is known about incidence, prevalence, and the effectiveness of treatment, including cost effectiveness'. The second, 'comparative assessments', is a mixed bag of performance, price, demographic data and Health Service indicators. And the third, 'a corporate view', is the familiar list of 'local people, GPs, providers and their clinical staff, other local agencies (FHSAs, LAs etc [*sic*]), Regions, and the NHSME' (NHSME, 1991b: 3). From these elements, by an unspecified and mysterious process, DHAs were to be able to 'establish local priorities' (*ibid.*).

The political difficulties

The confused and impenetrable nature of NHSE advice on purchasing is an inevitable consequence of its retreat into technical discussions when confronted with the political difficulties inherent in the exercise. It has encouraged what Hunter has described as the 'the curiously never-ending search for, and fascination with, technical solutions to what are at the end of the day political problems riven with value judgements that are not themselves susceptible to resolution through technical means or fixes' (Hunter, 1993: 8).

The early indications were that faced with this paradoxical situation purchasers on the whole avoided hard decisions and behaved with cautious incrementalism. In their analysis of the purchasing plans of 114 health authorities, Redmayne and Klein found that none of them adopted a scientific or cost-effectiveness approach to priority setting but settled with keeping the maximum number of people happy (Redmayne, 1992). Only 12 said they would either not buy or would limit the availability of specific forms of treatment and of these the researchers observed: 'These decisions represent merely symbolic gestures about the need to prioritize between different claims on resources rather than a serious attempt to address the issues' (quoted by Delamothe, 1992: 1241). What were the political difficulties which so inhibited purchasing agencies?

As the description of the Uncle Tom Cobley approach has shown, purchasing has vastly expanded the number of potential key players in the resource allocation game of the NHS. The effect, to quote Hunter once more, is that 'by increasing the visibility of a decision process, and by allowing many more individuals and groups access to it, the potential for conflict among key groups of decision makers [is] increased' (Hunter, 1991a: 20). Conflict is virtually assured by the absence of either any rules to ensure 'fair play' between the game players or any public means of conflict resolution. Such a situation encourages *ad hoc* decision making as the only recourse in the face of irresolvable pressures. This was clearly demonstrated in a worthy experiment by Southampton Health Authority to 'elucidate criteria for rationing' with the help of numerous experts. After much debate the members of the Health Authority announced that while 'grateful for the guidance of economists and philosophers' they were nonetheless 'in no doubt that their tough decisions on rationing could not be left to neat formulas', though no indication whatsoever was given as to how their decision would then be made (Cochrane, 1991: 1042).

Assuming that the political problem of how to make the decision about rationing is resolved, a further one awaits. Once a purchaser has decided the distribution and volume of health care it will buy for a given period, it faces the question of how far its decision is regarded as legitimate either by those who participated in the decision making process or by the citizenry at large, given the expectations generated by welfare state values. Southampton Health Authority, for one, was concerned about the likely public reception for any explicit rationing decision it might make, noting that:

> At present, it was agreed, the idea of people being denied health service is very foreign to most members of the public, and any progression down that route has to be understood and *ultimately approved by them*. (*ibid.*, emphasis added)

Traditionally, doctors have been able to legitimate their rationing of health care simply through the assertion of their professional values: their decisions are regarded as legitimate because they are impartial clinical judgements underpinned by the value of clinical freedom. Although some clinicians would acknowledge that other personal, ethical and legal factors can enter into this decision, they sensibly do not allow these to question the symbolic power of clinical freedom itself (Williams, 1988). The criticisms lately heaped upon the traditional form of rationing are a reflection of the values held by those seeking to displace the medical profession as the controlling agent in the allocation of health care resources and can be described as democratic and 'technical–rational'.

Much is made of the covert nature of the informal system of resource allocation arguing, as Maynard does for example, that the basis of the choices made is 'implicit, incoherent and inconsistent' (Society for Social Medicine, 1990: 188). It is generally assumed that implicit equals bad and explicit equals good because open decision making is a necessary part of democratic politics which, in turn, is self-legitimating. Thus in his eulogy to the Oregon experiment, Richard Smith, editor of the *British Medical Journal*, takes Sir Raymond Hoffenberg to task for suggesting that the limitation of services should be 'implicit, unstated, unwritten, unacknowledged – in the curious and not inhumane way in which such matters are managed in the United Kingdom'. Sir Raymond, he claims, 'has misread the Zeitgeist. Democracy in all it messy splendour is taking over everywhere', professions are suspect, paternalism is in decline and there is 'a rightful increase in demands for accountability'

(Smith, 1991: 1562). There is no recognition here that if democratic decision-making produces outcomes which strongly conflict with the expectations generated by the Health Service's universalistic values concerning access and treatment, the legitimacy of those outcomes may well be questioned both by groups and by individuals.

In this context the NHSE's views on the benefits of involving local citizens in purchasing decisions are politically naïve:

> Being responsive to local views will enhance the credibility of health authorities but, more importantly, is likely to result in services which are better suited to local needs and therefore more appropriate. There may of course be occasions when local views have to be over-ridden (for example, the weight of epidemiological, resource or other considerations) and in such circumstances, it is important that health authorities explain the reasons for their decisions. (NHSE, 1992a: 3)

Not only has it proved difficult to get local people involved (Donaldson, 1995) but also the results have still left purchasing agencies having to make the hard decisions without local support. Following a conference to review a strategy of involving 'local stakeholders', Southampton and South West Hampshire health commission concluded that 'only when ordinary people understand and accept that resources are finite will they accept that the role of the commission is legitimate' (Richards and Robinson, 1994: 25) – a situation which, given the state's continued emphasis on health care rights but not the limited NHS supply, is probably a long way off.

Closely linked to the democratic theme is the idea that purchasing decisions will be regarded as legitimate because they are arrived at by a process which is 'rational', 'technical' and 'scientific'. Health economists and supporters of formula funding are particularly prone to believe that because their methods have these characteristics, therefore they will be regarded by the public as a legitimate basis for deciding who will get what health care. Their assumption, clearly, is that the public is as rational as they are. Thus in discussing his resource allocation model based on public preferences for outcomes, Hadorn muses on the difficulty that regardless of the expressed preference of individuals or groups the general public often demands services for which there is little objective evidence of significant benefit. The answer must be a lack of information, he concludes, slightly edgily: 'once patients, physicians and payers are provided with information as to the lack of efficacy of treatments for most conditions, many of the motivations currently driving these actors to seek such treatments may evaporate' (Hadorn, 1991: 779). And, one is tempted to add, may not. Hunter, for one, has argued that the use of such methods will be counter-productive and that 'the introduction of half-understood technical devices on the part of policy makers and those not expert in such matters... will only serve to mystify and obfuscate discussions about priorities' (Hunter, 1993: 33).

Others are equally less sanguine, or less naïve, about the acceptability of the new purchasing arrangements to the populace at large and, referring to DHAs, maintain that 'the dangers of fragmentation on the purchasing side are at least as great as among providers' (Ham and Heginbotham, 1991a: 21). Rationing of itself is not a problem and can be easily achieved, writes Heginbotham, 'the issue is what is acceptable in a population or culture – ethically, economically, politically, socially and organisationally' (Heginbotham, 1992: 497). Once it is recognised that explicit rationing and the expectations created by the universalistic values of the NHS are mutually incompatible, and that the gap between the two cannot be bridged simply by characterising the purchasing process as democratic and rational, other political forms have to be found to resolve the conundrum. The choice is between changing the expectations through a redefinition of the British citizen's rights to welfare and changing the purchasing process. To date the focus has been upon the latter.

In addressing this problem, Klein argues that Health Authorities will 'have to start thinking seriously about the nature of their constituencies and how they can best generate support, professional and public, for their priorities' (Klein, 1991: 2). So here we have the idea of proactive purchasers, moving beyond the purchaser decision itself, to how that decision can then be sold, or legitimised, to their resident populations. It is an important change because it implies that the rationing decisions do not have to be democratic or rational, though they may be, but that they do have to be justified through conscious political action. As Strachan *et al.* point out, with a measure of understatement, this means that the chief executive of the DHA is then in the position of 'managing the political interface' because if public opinion is not successfully influenced in support of proposed changes, the pressure from local politicians and interest groups is likely 'to reduce the authority's effectiveness' (Strachan *et al.*, 1991: 15).

Given this web of political difficulties, how has the Health Service dealt with its new-found task of explicit rationing? In two respects the politicians have not dealt with it at all but simply exacerbated the difficulties, first, by raising public expectations of the NHS through The Patient's Charter and The Health of the Nation (HON) initiatives and, second, by creating new procedures through which patient discontent about their unmet expectations can be registered.

The Patient's Charter was introduced in April 1992 as the NHS contribution to the Citizen's Charter policy. It guaranteed seven existing rights, three new rights (on information availability, waiting times for treatment and complaints) and established nine National Charter Standards as benchmarks against which progress would be monitored (DoH, 1992a). Within a hegemony which instinctively applauds the expansion of social rights, such an initiative was bound to find fertile soil. In 1995 a new version called The Patient's Charter and You was published containing 26 *rights* ('which all patients will receive all the time') and 47 *expectations* ('these are standards of service which the NHS is aiming to achieve. Exceptional circumstances may sometimes prevent these standards being met') (DoH, 1995b: 4). As the industry of patients' rights has grown, so particularly deserving categories have been identified, notably pregnant women – The Maternity Charter – and children – The Children and Young People Charter. To sustain the impetus, monitoring arrangements have been introduced and, beginning in 1994, the results published annually as part of the Citizen's Charter under the not unprovocative title of The NHS Performance Guide. Readers of the reports are encouraged to make comparisons of the performance of individual Trusts on three categories of patient rights: choice, prompt service and information.

The effect of The Patient's Charter has been to create new areas of patient demand, politicise them, and construct new systems for measuring the state's ability, or inability, to meet that demand. In effect, the state has made a social rights rod with which to beat its own back. Less specific but nonetheless providing general encouragement for the spiral of health care demand has been The Health of the Nation initiative. It is strangely ironic that in his foreword to the Green Paper on HON, William Waldegrave, then Secretary of State for Health, introduced his new policy with the statement: 'resources which can be devoted to health care will always be finite in the face of infinite demand. Setting priorities is therefore essential' (DoH, 1991: 3). Yet from a priority-setting exercise HON rapidly moved to become an instrument of demand expansion. The subsequent White Paper, subtitled 'A Strategy for Health in England', announced that it was:

> only the start of a continuing process of identifying priority objectives, setting targets and monitoring and reviewing progress. Over time new objectives and targets will be set, adding to or replacing those in this White Paper. (DoH, 1992b: 3)

Fuelled by the hegemonic urge for social rights growth, it was the target setting which rapidly became the driving force of the policy rather than any notion of making difficult choices for the disposal of 'finite resources'. Key areas were identified (coronary heart disease, cancers, mental illness, HIV/AIDS and sexual health, accidents), monitoring protocols discussed, implementation procedures promulgated, and national indicators and information requirements (existing and proposed) explored (DoH, 1992c). A bureaucratic star was born and it shone radiantly. Its short-term political utility was undeniable: it gave the Department of Health a strategy, the threatened public health profession a role (Salter, 1993a), and numerous health interest groups a convenient lobbyist's vehicle for the inevitable call for more resources. Its progress reports are respectably statistical and provide excellent platforms for advertising the public relations side of HON: new developments (for example, Health of the Young Nation initiative), conferences, newsletters, alliances (for example with industry and the voluntary sector), working groups and task forces (DoH, 1993b, 1995c). With the backing of a Cabinet committee HON also acts as a useful resource in the internecine warfare that is part of interdepartmental relationships in government by requiring the cooperation of other departments.

The effect of this considerable activity is that the Department not only has an explicit health strategy but one that is highly visible, quantifiable and readily accountable. It encourages the population to reflect that, on a variety of known indicators, it should be getting healthier and, if it is not, the state is failing in its self-appointed task. If HON targets are not met, then the public can legitimately feel aggrieved that its right to, and expectation of, improved health has also not been fulfilled. (A progress report on HON by the National Audit Office showed 'good' progress towards only 40 per cent of the set goals – National Audit Office, 1996.) Once again, the demand side has been given an extra twist.

And if those expectations do go unfulfilled then, with impeccable logic, the state has also sought to streamline the way in which the consequent discontent can be registered on the unhappy NHS purchasers and providers. Both the Code of Practice on Openness in the NHS and the new NHS complaints procedures promulgated by the NHSE following *Being Heard*, the report of the Wilson Committee (DoH, 1995a), are at pains to point out that they are building on progress already made through The Patient's Charter (NHSE, 1995a: 2; NHSE, 1995b: 2). Driven by the relentless imperatives of The Patient's Charter, both contain a comprehensive list of actions, procedures and good practice which are mandatory, which will be monitored and, the intention is, enforced through the accountability line of Health Authorities, regional offices and NHSE. As the standards and targets of the The Patient's Charter and The Health of the Nation become more ambitious and refined, so the likelihood of unmet expectations will increase and the impact of disenchanted patients will be legitimised and concentrated by the new openness and complaints procedures.

At the national level, therefore, there is a continuing sense of ambiguity in official pronouncements as politicians fight shy of confronting the powder-keg of the demand–supply mismatch in state welfare in general and health care in particular. The long-standing policy of not making choices has produced what the House of Commons Health Committee has termed 'priority overload' as the many *ad hoc* priorities issued to the NHS have mounted (Health Committee of the House of Commons, 1995a: xvii). Yet although the Committee might inveigh against what it described as 'wish lists', it also felt obliged to admit that 'there is no such thing as a correct set of priorities, or even a correct way of setting priorities' (which rather let the government off the hook) (*ibid.*: xxiii). The government's reaction to the Committee was to cultivate the ambiguity further. First, it recognised that: 'budgets will always be finite while demand is potentially open-ended. There will always be a gap between all we wish to do and all that we can. Setting priorities is a fact of life' (DoH, 1995a: 1). Second, it distanced itself from the act of rationing but added a significant caveat:

> The DoH does not seek to instruct local purchasers on what procedures they should or should not purchase, or under what circumstances. However, we would be concerned if there were blanket restrictions on a specific service where there was no provision for clinical need to be demonstrated in individual cases. (*ibid.*: 9)

So while the DoH recognises that rationing has to take place, if a particular service is not provided locally, it is not the fault of the DoH.

Further confusion has been caused by the use of the term 'priority-setting' as a euphemism for 'target-setting'. Hence the annual NHSE circular *Priorities and Planning: Guidance for the NHS* says nothing about how purchasing agencies are to make choices given limited resources and a great deal about how they must achieve an ever-growing list of 'baseline requirements and objectives', 'medium term priorities' and 'milestones' (NHSE, 1995c). The delicious irony then is that the only central guidance on priorities has the effect of making the task of rationing the existing purchaser resources more, rather than less, difficult.

So long as the political ploy of studied equivocation works at the national level, or at least does no noticeable damage, it is unlikely to be replaced by anything more positive or risky. Hence, while such illustrious sources as the Royal College of Physicians (Royal College of Physicians, 1995), the editor of the *British Medical Journal* (Smith, 1995a), and professional NHS commentators (Healthcare 2000, 1995) may call for national debate and action on priority setting, the politicians remain unmoved.

Where the only central guidance is a policy of *laissez-faire*, but where the gap between the demand for and supply of health care is becoming ever wider, purchasing agencies have lately begun to arrive at their own *ad hoc* solutions. In some cases this has meant the curtailment of treatment of such conditions as varicose veins, non-malignant lumps and bumps, wisdom teeth, tatoos, and *in vitro* fertilisation (IVF) – conditions where there is a clinical, though not necessarily a social, argument for rationing to take place and where the conditions are not life-threatening. For the most part, the criteria used to identify such conditions are not explicit but can be best described as 'clinical commonsense'. Some Authorities such as Salisbury (Chadda, 1993) and Salford (Healthcare 2000, 1995: 38) have sought to develop methods for the priority ranking of treatments. But they are the exceptions rather than the rule. The political sensitivity of this kind of low-key rationing exercise and the opposition it has aroused has varied, largely depending on the local circumstances. However, where the rationing involves a condition which is life-threatening (and which would previously have been handled covertly through the exercise of clinical judgement) the political fall-out can be considerable. Hence, the decision by Cambridge and Huntingdon health commission not to fund a second bone-marrow transplant for a child (known as 'child B') with leukaemia was taken to the Court of Appeal where it was upheld. The commission had an explicit and what they maintained was a rational policy of not funding new, experimental and unevaluated treatments for children with malignant diseases except in the context of ethically approved trials (Chadda, 1995). This did not save it from the media circus and public opprobrium.

The other purchasing agencies have so far been spared exposure to the full weight of the hegemonic values of state welfare. Unlike the Health Authority purchasers, GP Fundholders (and FHSAs up to 1996) incorporate the traditional, covert gatekeeping function and, as yet, have not faced the Health Authorities' political problems of explicit rationing, the legitimation of priorities and the control of consumer demand. However, it is debatable whether this happy situation will survive the expansion of Fundholder numbers, the increase in the list of elective treatment they are responsible for funding, and downward pressure on the financial incentives available to Fundholders. As money is progressively transferred from Health Authority to Fundholder budgets, so there is an objective demand for Fundholders to be uniformly financed according to a common formula rather than according to their historical referral patterns given the well-documented differences between Fundholders' *per capita* incomes. The cumulative effect of these changes is likely to be that GP Fundholders will have to make the same kind of rationing choices within a fixed budget as Health Authorities already do but without the financial leeway enjoyed by the earlier waves of Fundholders. Furthermore, as the spotlight of public concern about purchasing is progressively transferred along with the funding from Health Authorities to Fundholders, so their potential vulnerability will increase. While the process of covert rationing using clinical judgement will no doubt continue for a time, it will be more difficult to sustain as the public becomes more aware that Fundholders' are operating within fixed budgets. If and when the ideological power of clinical judgement as a rationing agent is undermined, the key political issue then becomes one of whether Fundholders would be prepared to act as the mechanism for explicit rationing.

Conclusions

It is perhaps ironic that the very reforms which were intended to use a market approach to the NHS to transfer power from the doctors to the consumers are now set to reinforce the influence of one part of the medical profession, the GPs, as a result of the politics of purchasing. Of itself, the new function of purchasing has had no direct effect on the central political problem of the NHS, that of the control of the demand for health care, because it has not so far addressed the issue of how to stabilise, redirect or reduce, the expectations created by the values of the welfare state hegemony. Instead it has taken those expectations as given, acknowledged that they exceed the available supply of health care, and then either ignored the consequent dilemma or sought to construct an explicit mechanism for deciding how to meet some expectations and not meet others. In so doing, it has become enmeshed in a complex political game where a predominant characteristic is one of puzzlement that the rules are either not known or constantly evolving, that the organisational components of purchasing are changing, and that the number of officially recommended gameplayers is virtually unlimited.

This uncertainty can be understood as a series of interlinked political problems which derive from the control of demand issue inherent in the Health Service since its foundation in 1948. Historically, the issue has been dealt with covertly by the medical profession through the use of informal rationing mechanisms which, because they were supported by the full power of the ideology of clinical freedom, remained largely unquestioned by the general public. However, the sound political principle of letting sleeping dogs lie became increasingly untenable as public expectations of the NHS continued to rise, resulting in a questioning not so much of the clinical rationing process itself as of its effects: access to health care and, in particular, waiting times.

With the introduction of the 1991 reforms the formal responsibility for dealing with the demand–supply mismatch in the NHS became the domain of the purchasing agencies. They are given a fixed budget to decide who gets what health care. Given public expectations of the NHS, the political problems faced by purchasers were several. First, the duties, basis of funding and operational methods of the three agencies (DHAs and FHSAs – now merged to form Health Authorities – and GP Fundholders) were different and inconsistent. Their inter-organisational relationships were fluid and frequently competitive and territorial disputes were not uncommon. But the key difference between them, and hence the nature of the political problems faced by each, was that while FHSAs and GP Fundholders automatically incorporated the traditional gatekeepers to the NHS (the GPs) the DHAs, certainly initially, did not and therefore sought to develop their own rationing mechanisms. The formal merger of DHAs and FHSAs to form the new Health Authorities did not of itself impact on this issue insofar as the Authorities still have to carry out the separate DHA and FHSA purchasing functions in secondary and primary care.

As the largest purchasing agency with the proclaimed role of 'champions of the people', DHAs had a visibility denied to the other two agencies. In constructing a decision-making procedure for allocating resources, they were expected to adhere to the open and comprehensive consultative procedures recommended by the NHSE and take into consideration the views of public health physicians, health economists, consumers, providers and so on as they went about the business of identifying the population's 'health care needs'. What neither they nor their successor Health Authorities have, however, is any guidance on the means to resolve the inescapable conflict between these different viewpoints. Who is right and who is wrong? Inevitably different Health Authorities will find different ways of solving the riddle.

Having reached what, by definition, will be an idiosyncratic decision about the rationing of the available resources, each Health Authority then faces the third and intractable political problem of legitimating that decision to the local populace, at which point the clash with the citizens' health care rights and expectations becomes manifest. The evidence on the effects of that clash supports Mechanic's claim that:

> Explicit rationing is inevitably unstable because of the ability of small groups to evoke public sympathy and support in contesting government decision making. Those who care deeply but are denied access will inevitably challenge the explicit judgement through the mass media and in other ways, undermining support for purchasing decisions and pushing the health system towards more flexible implicit approaches. (Mechanic, 1995: 1658)

Examples of this phenemonon abound. North East Thames RHA's advice to DHAs to curtail treatment for varicose veins, non-malignant lumps and bumps, wisdom teeth, tattoos, and *in vitro* fertilisation produced a furore (Dixon and Welch, 1991) as did the North Western public health director's assertion that there should be checks on drugs prescribed to 'hopeless cases' of terminally ill patients

(Moore, 1992a) and the decision of the Scottish Office not to fund IVF centrally (Limb, 1993).

A key question is whether purchasing agencies will receive overt government support for explicit rationing. Given the electoral cost of taking a public stand against the principles of comprehensive health care embodied in the NHS, this is an unlikely course for any politician to take: witness the speed with which Steven Dorrell, the then Secretary of State for Health, rejected the report from the Healthcare 2000 committee where recommendations were made concerning the inevitability of rationing (Healthcare 2000, 1995). In so doing he was reflecting the dominant reaction one would expect when an hegemony as emotive and powerful as the welfare state is directly challenged. (One eminent observer described the report as 'barking mad' (Maynard, 1995).) In an earlier example when Oxford Health Authority sought to place explicit limits on its sterilisation services, the Secretary of State William Waldegrave interestingly supported informal rationing when he took the view that while it is acceptable for doctors to make choices between which patients to treat (presumably on the grounds of clinical judgement), Health Authorities are not entitled to make policy decisions excluding categories of patients (Ewart, 1991: 19).

Assuming there is no clear national lead, Health Authorities will be left to fight a series of local ideological conflicts to convince their catchment populations that both priority-setting itself, and its outcomes, are acceptable. It is unlikely to be a simple case, as Smith would have us believe, of 'following the Oregonians into the sunlight' through the application of democracy, reason, frankness and goodwill (Smith, 1991: 1562). Any attempt to challenge the expectations embedded in the NHS values of comprehensive health care will inevitably arouse substantial opposition and will require Health Authorities to exhibit a high level of political skill. How far their corporate contracts with the NHSE and the increasing use of target-setting will allow them the appropriate freedom of manoeuvre to demonstrate such skills is as yet an unanswered question. What is certain is that any Health Authority strategy for dealing with the demand–supply mismatch in health care will require the cooperation of GPs as the gatekeepers to the NHS.

For the future, it is probable that some of the foregoing political problems will be redirected as a result of the growth of GP Fundholders and their shouldering of a greater proportion of the purchasing, and therefore of the rationing, responsibility. But what is unknown is how far they will be willing, and able, to use clinical judgement as the means for legitimising their decisions. Once it is clear to the public that GPs are the financial as well as the clinical gatekeepers to the NHS and that resource considerations form part of the decision to refer, GPs will find themselves under quite new political pressures.

3

Providing

Introduction

The stated objective of the 1991 reforms was to create a simple functional divide between purchasers and providers. Purchasers were to identify the health care needs of their populations and commission the services required, providers were to concentrate on the efficient delivery of their contracts with purchasers. Theoretically at least, this arrangement means that power, responsibility and the levers for change in the NHS lie with the purchasing agencies. One might therefore be forgiven for assuming that it is purchasers alone who have to deal with the Health Service's fundamental political problem of excess demand for health care and that providers would be able to shelter behind their contractual dependence on purchasers.

It is a tribute to the limited impact of formal policy innovation on the fundamental politics of the NHS that the 1991 reforms have done nothing to reduce the exposure of providers to the demand–supply mismatch in health care. Purchasing agencies may be experiencing the novel political difficulties of the overt rationing of supply but this has not diminished the long-established need for the management of demand by those who provide the service. What has changed is the way in which this reconciliation between patient rights and health care resources takes place within provider organisations.

This chapter explores the extent to which the changes in the context and organisation of provider Trusts has altered the relationship between their internal power structures and their handling of excess demand. (The provider issue in primary care is dealt with in Chapter 4.) It begins by examining the traditional method of rationing employed by the medical profession and the functional basis of their power in the NHS. This constitutes a political baseline which all policy innovation has, perforce, to recognise. Second, it analyses the plurality of accountability systems within which Trusts are situated and their effect on Trust behaviour. This then brings the chapter to the critical question of demand control under the new order: to what extent have the changes in provider organisation had an impact on clinicians' handling of demand?

The management of demand

With the foundation of the NHS in 1948, citizens were given the right to comprehensive health care which was to be free at the point of delivery. The absence of a price mechanism in this arrangement, and hence of any cost to the patient of registering his/her right, meant that an alternative method was required to regulate the relationship between the demand for and supply of health care. After a suitable period of bargaining, the medical profession offered its services. It would use its professional authority as a means of governing the exercise of citizens' health care rights provided that, in return, doctors were given clinical, economic and political autonomy within the structure of the NHS.

Autonomy is the ability of a particular group to set the terms on which it interacts with its environment. The more it is able to do so, the more autonomy it has. The 1858 Medical Act had already given medicine clinical autonomy: the right to regulate its own professional affairs. With the 1946 NHS Act that basic autonomy was extended to include the economic and political spheres. Before the creation of the NHS, the income of the medical profession was based on a fee-for-service system which allowed its monopoly position in the health care market to be translated into tangible economic benefits. As a condition of its participation in the new policy, the profession gained a guarantee from the state that this market advantage would be incorporated into the contractual arrangements between doctors and the NHS: hospital doctors became permanent salaried employees of the state, a professionally controlled merit award system recognised the special position of consultants and GPs remained self-employed but with an assured contract and income. At the same time, there was formal recognition by the state of the right of NHS doctors to engage in private practice and continue to exploit their market position if they so desired. Thus the profession translated its existing economic advantages into a secure, state-sponsored system of economic autonomy (Klein, 1989: Ch. 1). Also, now that the patient's ability to pay was no longer a relevant factor, the economic constraint on clinical decision making was removed and the profession's clinical autonomy was enhanced accordingly (Elston, 1991: 67).

Clinical decisions are also decisions about the disposal of resources because, as Calman observes, 'in most instances it is the diagnosis which will determine the resources required' (Calman, 1994a: 1141). It follows logically, therefore, that acceptance of the principle of clinical autonomy is also an acceptance of the right of doctors to dispose of resources as they think fit. Any other view would be an infringement of the clinical autonomy principle. Effectively this gave the medical profession political autonomy within the NHS system; a principle recognised with unconscious irony by the report *Management Arrangements for the Reorganised Health Service* which heralded the management reorganisation of 1974:

> The distinguishing characteristic of the NHS is that to do their work properly consultants and general practitioners must have clinical autonomy, so that they can be fully responsible for the treatment they prescribe to their patients. It follows that these doctors and dentists work as each others equals and that *they are their own managers*. In ethics and law they are accountable to their patients for the care they prescribe and *they cannot be held accountable* to the NHS authorities for the quality of their clinical judgements so long as they act within the broad limits of acceptable medical practice and within policy for the use of resources. (DHSS, 1972: para 1.18; quoted by Stacey, 1984: 13, emphasis added)

As Klein observes, 'implicit in the structure of the NHS 'was the bargain between the state and the medical profession which ensured that 'while central government controlled the budget, doctors controlled what happened within that budget' (Klein, 1989: 82). The state would manage the overall parameters of the supply side leaving doctors to manage the intricacies of the supply–demand interface.

Under the fee-for-service system which had governed the doctor–patient relationship before the arrival of the NHS, the management of this interface had been facilitated by the cost constraints experienced by patients and by their consequent assumption that the service available to them as individuals was finite. With the removal of this constraint by the universalistic and open-ended nature of NHS provision, the only justifiable limit on the supply of health care to a particular patient under the new regime was that it was not clinically necessary. This caveat excepted, NHS values assumed the supply to be infinite. How were hospital doctors to carry out their crucial political function of reconciling the demand–supply relationship whilst remaining loyal to the utopian promises of the NHS? What they required was a mechanism with a private and a public reality. Privately it should ration resources; publicly it should be the vehicle for purely clinical decisions. Waiting lists were the natural solution.

Waiting lists are a temporal extension to the private professional world of the clinician. Traditionally they have been regarded as purely medical territory which others enter at their peril. It is instructive to explore how they work since it is this long-established practice which is at the heart of the profession's power to control demand. Taking surgery as an example, each surgeon has a waiting list composed of two sequential queues for out-patient consultations and in-patient treatment. Each queue has a fast and a slow stream (urgent and non-urgent patients). In theory, the admission to each queue and the designation as urgent or non-urgent within each queue are decisions made by the surgeon on the basis of his/her clinical judgement. In practice, the waiting list is used to structure and manipulate patient demand to satisfy numerous non-clinical criteria – including the criterion of available resources. Decisions not to refer for in-patient treatment may be guided by the patient's social characteristics such as age in the case of renal dialysis (Halper, 1989) and coronary care (Dudley and Burns, 1992) or whether he/she is a smoker or non-smoker in the case of cardiac surgery (Hughes and Griffiths, 1996; more generally see Charney *et al.*, 1989). Within the in-patient queue, resequencing regularly takes place when patients are selected for operation one week in advance 'taking into account a number of criteria including case mix for variety to satisfy a registrar's training requirements or research interest, to fit with the theatre and staff availability, as well as urgency and the time the individual patients have been in the queue' (West, 1993: 48). None of this is public knowledge as it would undermine the myth of clinical impartiality.

Publicly, waiting lists have the added advantage to the specialist that they can be used to massage, as well as restrict, demand and so enhance his/her professional reputation if required. Changes in the admission threshold and in the operation and/or discharge rate can dramatically increase the size of the waiting list and so demonstrate to managers, colleagues or referring GPs the apparent demand for the clinician's services and, who knows, perhaps even encourage demand for his/her private practice (*ibid.*: 59). In the absence of a price mechanism, waiting lists denote desirability and prestige (Pope, 1992: 79).

The division between the private and public reality of waiting lists is thus politically and professionally functional and a necessary component of the bargain between medicine and the state. It enables the practical reconciliation of the political task of demand control with the professional privileges of clinical, economic and political autonomy. Because it is so central to the operation of the NHS, it not only endows the medical profession with unrivalled power but creates a rigidity in the system which any putative change must address if it is not to create instability in the Health Service's political functions. It is a central tenet of the NHS ideology that doctors make their decisions purely on the basis of clinical criteria uninfluenced by economic and political factors and it is this characteristic which, in the eyes of patients, renders their decisions impartial, legitimate and acceptable. If this were not the case then the ability of doctors to control the expectations of patients would be much diminished. There is thus an automatic linkage between the political function of demand management and professional autonomy: to change one is to change the other.

Yet since the early 1980s the state has expended considerable effort in promoting changes in NHS provision which do not address this fundamental issue. Faced with increasing evidence of the demand–supply mismatch in health care, the state has focused exclusively on the supply side of the equation and has consistently taken the view that the problem should be dealt with by improving the efficiency and effectiveness with which health care is delivered. Commencing with *The NHS Management Inquiry* (Griffiths Report) in 1983, the general policy has been that consultants 'must accept the management responsibility which goes with clinical freedom' and the resources which are dispensed as a result of their clinical decisions (Department of Health and Social Security [DHSS], 1983a, 19). At the same time, a new class of general managers was created to drive the various intiatives which grew out of the policy, establish a cost-conscious environment and provide greater direction to the management of hospitals. The intention was that tying clinical decision making to fixed budgets would lead both to greater efficiency and to an automatic rationing of supply.

There was no good reason why the medical profession should cooperate with this policy as there was every chance that it would alter the nature of their professional autonomy within the NHS. Because the profession was too powerful to be told what to do, the DHSS resorted to persuasion and attempted seduction – neither of which worked. Attempts were made throughout the 1980s to facilitate the implementation of the Griffiths recommendations with the help of the Management Budgeting and Resource Management initiatives which aimed to provide clinicians with computerised financial data systems to aid their decision-making, but clinicians' interest remained largely unengaged. The 1986 DHSS review of Management Budgeting concluded that it had failed principally through concentrating overmuch on the technical aspects of budgeting at the expense of winning the support and commitment of key personnel: managers, clinicians, and finance officers (Young, 1986). So Resource Management was introduced in its stead as a wider approach that would emphasise 'medical and nursing ownership of the system' and would generate extensive clinical as well as financial information (DHSS, 1986b). But this also proved to be a white elephant.

The use of information systems as a device to tempt clinicians into the parlour of managerial responsibility was always likely to fail because it was not accompanied by incentives to offset the disadvantages of such a move. In their study of the introduction of general management Harrison and his associates observed, whilst quoting a senior hospital doctor that 'the idea that many clinicians would be interested in taking on time consuming management posts was "one of the serious fallacies of Griffiths"' (Harrison *et al.*, 1989: 11). In part the shift to Resource Management recognised this issue but the suggested solution was more training or a vague reference to an unspecified organisational change. Thus in their interim evaluation of Resource Management, Packwood and his associates write, 'It appears a common experience that the scale of cultural change involved was initially underestimated. Training has to be provided in step with the introduction of the new information technology' (Packwood *et al.*, 1990: 254). However, the offer of training had little appeal when measured against the advantages already enjoyed by doctors of money, status and power. Of those who ventured into the field of general management itself, most decided it was not for them. Between 1985 and 1991 the number of doctors heading the management of districts and hospitals halved from 120 to 58. Lack of remuneration is cited as one reason, the loss of private practice and the hostility of medical colleagues as others (Millar, 1991).

While doctors could choose whether or not they engaged with the post-Griffiths drive to improve efficiency in the NHS, the new cadre of general managers enjoyed no such luxury. They were accountable not only for their own performance but also for that of the organisation as a whole; and it was largely the resource-allocating decisions of clinicians that determined the latter. General managers were thus in the paradoxical position where they were held accountable for the aggregate decisions of a group (doctors) whose professional ideology, founded on a high-level bargain with the state, insisted that its members should only be accountable to each other, if at all, and certainly not to managers. The effect was to give managers considerable responsibility but little power.

The power rivalry which consequently developed between managers and clinicians is sustained and fuelled by their opposing cultures. Hunter sums up the basic difference thus: 'The concern of doctors to do what is best for the individual patient may conflict with the need to set priorities within services, to maintain expenditure within agreed limits, and to maximise the benefits of service to the population served' (Hunter, 1991b: 443). The right of the clinician to focus exclusively on the interests of a single patient without reference to the commonweal is legitimised in principle by the concept of clinical freedom and in practice by the fact that all consultants in the NHS have equal status and none has authority over another. In its pure form, this value position leads inexorably to the belief that clinicians should not actively participate in hospital management as this could compromise their medical judgement (Chant, 1984). Nor is this the extreme view of a small minority. A recent survey by the NHS Executive's Training Division found that 70 per cent of doctors rejected management as part of their everyday clinical practice (Turner, 1995: 13). The two opposing cultures effectively create two organisations in one with the result, as Pettigrew and his colleagues observe, that the NHS 'is characterised by a large number of "street level bureaucrats" and by a shadow professional organisation located within bureaucratic structures, eroding still further the capacity for "rational" decision making' (Pettigrew *et al.*, 1988: 309). Reluctant bedfellows, the differences and hostility between them are unavoidable and well-documented (see for example National Health Service Training Authority, 1987; Scrivens, 1987).

It is, however, an unequal rivalry because while the political function of doctors is central to the existence of the NHS, that of managers is not. Of themselves, managers can have little effect on the demand–supply relationship in health care. As a result, when the tension between them spills into conflict in the public arena, it is almost invariably the clinicians who receive the backing of the Secretary of State for Health and the manager who suffers. To take a high-profile example, John Spiers, who in 1994 was obliged to resign as chairman of Brighton Health Care Trust after consultants passed a vote of no confidence in him, observed:

> When I speak to managers around the country the message I hear is the same. They say: 'Look what happened to you in Brighton – we don't dare take them [clinicians] on'. (Waters, 1995: 13)

For managers, there is no escape from the continuing tension between their accountability for policy implementation and the blocking power of doctors (Thompson, 1987).

The web of accountability

But when the internal market reforms were launched in 1991, the public rhetoric was that they marked a distinctive shift in the way NHS care was delivered and a qualitative break with the past. *Working for Patients* describes how NHS Hospital Trusts were to have a range of powers and freedoms not available to the then existing Health Authorities:

> NHS Hospital Trusts will be empowered by statute to employ staff; to enter into contracts both to provide services and to buy in services and supplies with others; and to raise income within the scope set by the Health and Medicine's Act 1988. (DoH, 1989a: 23)

Each hospital's assets was to be vested in its Trust and it was to be free to use its assets to provide health care, dispose of assets, have an interest-bearing debt equal to the value of its assets, and to retain surpluses and build up reserves. At the same time it was free to borrow money from the private financial market subject to the constraint imposed by its External Financing Limit (EFL) (*ibid.*: 25). As an independent trader within the public sector, each Trust would be able to determine its own destiny.

Within the new provider organisations, there was the clear implication that the new policy would lead to a shift in power in favour of the managers. Four years into the internal market, we find that the

Audit Commission at least was convinced that such a redistribution had occurred following the implementation of the organisational changes detailed in *Working for Patients*:

> Managers now have more control over the employment of staff and the management of capital. They have taken over the employment of consultants from regional or district health authorities and they can negotiate local pay and conditions for a wide range of staff. They can use retained surpluses or Treasury capital within their external financing limit and they can enter into arrangements that use private sector capital such as operating leases or joint ventures, provided the risk is equitably shared. And it is now more acceptable to consider sub-contracting services, leaving managers free to concentrate on core activities. (Audit Commission, 1994a: 3)

It is, however, unwise to equate an improvement in managerial capacity with an increase in managerial power.

Trusts are situated within a web of contractual and bureaucratic accountabilities which severely restrict both the freedoms technically available to them as organisations and the ability of their managers to take advantage of their new decision making capacities. Their problems begin with the fact that they have no distinct legal identity and hence no clear foundation on which to bargain for their putative independence (Long and Salter, 1994). Legally they are companies, not 'Trusts', but unlike most other companies they are created by statute and defined as 'statutory corporations'. This means they are neither regulated nor protected by the Companies Acts 1985–9, nor by the regulations made by the Department of Trade and Industry under those Acts and the whole body of company law does not apply to them. As statutory corporations, Trusts have no powers other than those given to them by the statute that brought them into existence. They are therefore regulated by the NHS and Community Care Act 1990 and the statutory instrument 'SI 1990 no. 2024, The National Health Service Trusts (membership and procedure) regulations 1990' and each is empowered by a separate statutory instrument which constitutes its establishment order.

The legal powers of Trusts defined in the Act and these regulations are very general and very few. There is no attempt to give them the list of powers usually contained in a limited company's object clause. Their legal capacity to act as trading agents in the open market is therefore severely, and, one must assume, deliberately restricted and any pursuance of the normal company's range of market activities is bound to render Trusts *ultra vires*. A final confirmation of Trusts as pretend-companies playing an unreal game of NHS monopoly lies in the legal concept of 'an NHS contract' (a contract between NHS bodies) which the 1990 Act expressly states 'is not a contract in law' (section 4[3]). In any contractual dispute, Trusts are obliged to seek recourse not from the law but from arbitration carried out by a bureaucratic arm of the National Health Service Executive (NHSE).

Lacking legal independence and clear statutory powers, Trusts have no alternative but to work within bureaucratic systems of accountability which they do not have the power to challenge. To this extent the NHS has not changed. What has changed is that although greater operational control may have been devolved to provider organisations, their upward lines of accountability are more numerous and more exacting than before. Broadly speaking, the systems of accountability fall into two categories: contract- and non-contract-based systems.

Trusts engage in contracts with four types of purchasing agencies for the delivery of different services: Health Authorities and GP Fundholders (patient services), University Medical Schools and Postgraduate Deans (undergraduate and postgraduate medical education), Working Paper 10 consortia of employing Trusts (nursing and other non-medical education) and NHS research and development funding bodies (research). In all cases the contracts are becoming more detailed and specific in their requirements, more careful and systematic in their monitoring of performance and more prepared to use sanctions in the event of inappropriate outcomes. As the purchasing agencies intensify their search for increased value for money, so they are placing provider Trusts under greater and conflicting accountability pressures. In effect, Trusts are competing for business in what are now the four markets of patient services, medical education, nursing and other non-medical education, and research. Whereas pre-1991 the demands of these arenas were imperfectly registered, linked to funding only in a notional fashion, and scarcely regarded as accountable at all, they are now contract and budget based and themselves subject to more rigorous monitoring from the higher echelons of the NHS. For provider hospitals, the new systems of accountability are steadily diminishing traditional areas of flexibility in their organisation of their affairs.

The consequences are becoming particularly evident in the burgeoning tension between the demands, on the one hand, of Health Authorities and GP Fundholders and, on the other, of Medical Schools and Postgraduate Deans. As their contracting expertise has developed, Health Authority and GP Fundholders have become ever

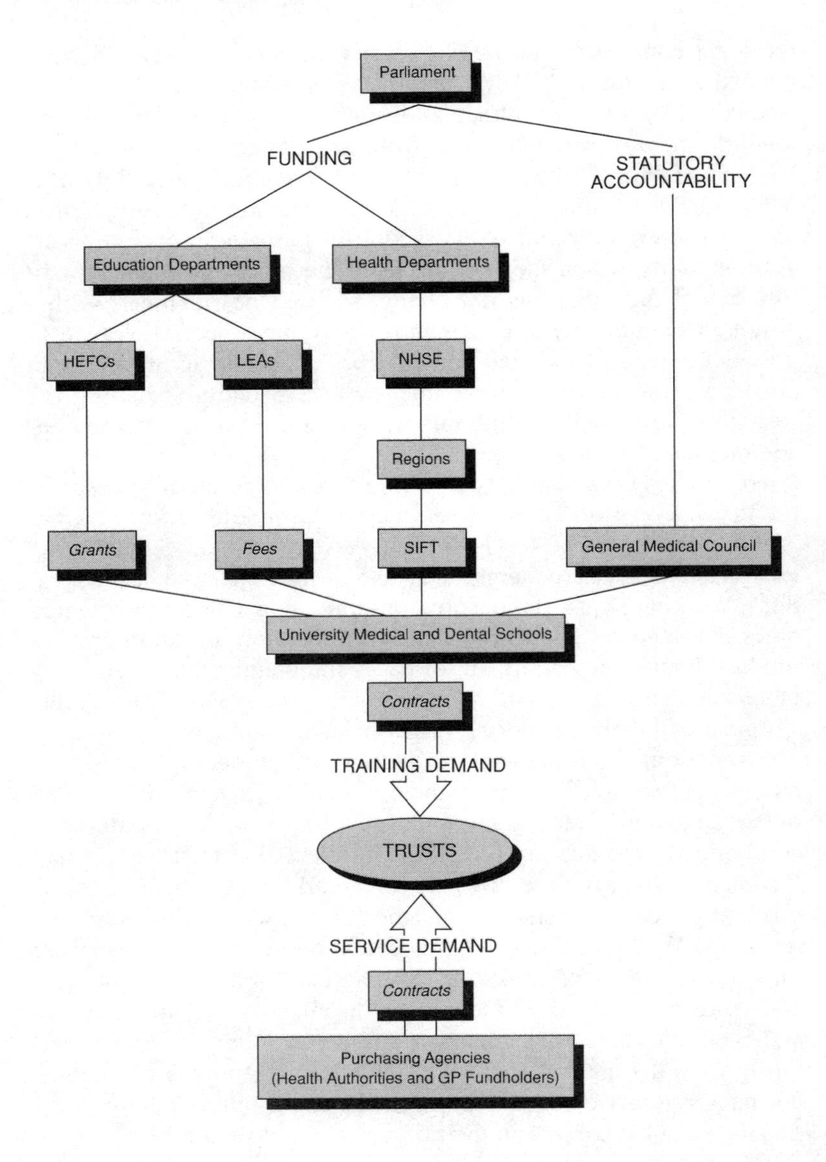

Figure 3.1 Undergraduate medical education

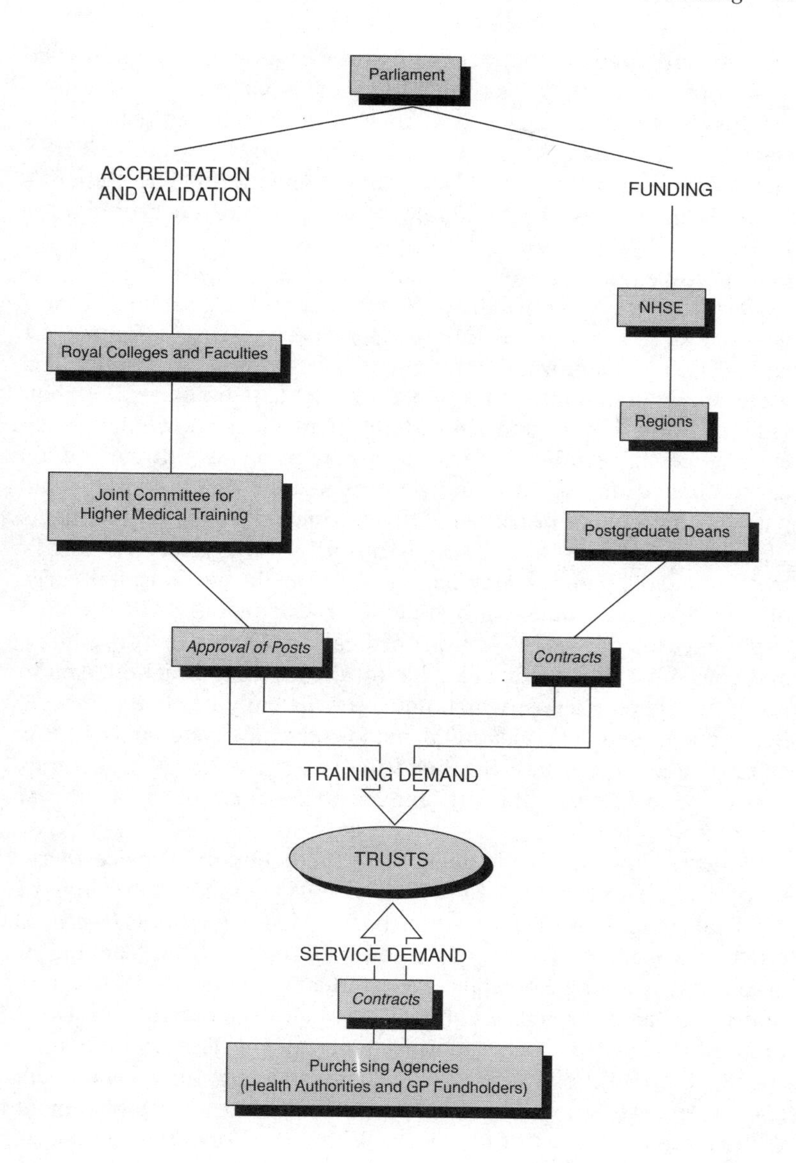

Figure 3.2 Postgraduate and continuing medical education

more specific in their contracts with providers about the quantity and quality of service they require and in their monitoring of what they get for their money. In the case of Health Authorities there is the sustaining impetus of their own corporate contracts with the NHSE and, within these, the highly visible demands of The Patient's Charter. In the case of Fundholders the pressure on providers is fuelled by an ancient, and until now unabated frustration, with the unresponsiveness of hospital consultants to GPs' needs.

At the same time Medical Schools and Postgraduate Deans generate a contract-based training demand on Trusts (Figures 3.1 and 3.2). Doctors in training require a diverse range of hospital, and increasingly community, experiences to enable them to develop their clinical skills through the application of medical knowledge. Such experiences have to be structured as part of an overall curriculum and delivered through a training infrastructure which overlaps and parallels the system of service delivery. Inevitably the requirements of service delivery and medical training will differ. To satisfy training needs, patients may have to be brought into hospital early, or their discharge delayed, a student's rota adapted to incorporate experience of the less common medical conditions or procedures, and consultant time made available for the teaching function. And to all of this there is a cost which until very recently has been ignored. Service and medical education demands have always co-existed in a state of uneasy tension, but historically diffuse lines of accountability have allowed the differences to be fudged and informal compromises reached.

Undergraduate medical education is funded by the Service Increment for Teaching (SIFT) which is NHS money allocated to Medical Schools on a *per capita* basis. Medical schools use it to contract the undergraduate education they require from teaching or associated teaching hospitals. Postgraduate (junior doctor) education is financed through a contract between the Postgraduate Dean (a joint NHS-University appointment) and a Trust which may specify the facilities to be provided, the standards to be achieved, and the non-variation of the hospital's junior doctor establishment without the agreement of the Dean. Within the Trust, the contract is managed and the budget controlled by the Clinical Tutor, a consultant who is both an employee of the Trust and, through a separate contract, accountable to the Dean. So, technically at least, this arrangement allows training demand to be very specifically directed at the local Trust level. It is reinforced by the Trust's accountability to a further set of external agencies, the medical Royal Colleges, which increasingly act in concert with the Postgraduate Dean. Although not based on an explicit contract, the conditions and sanctions of the relationship between Trusts and Colleges are sufficiently precise to be said to constitute an implicit contract.

Most medical posts in hospitals form part of the system of medical education in the sense that they are occupied either by students (junior doctors) or teachers (consultants). In order to be regarded as a legitimate part of that system, however, they have to be 'approved' by the relevant Royal College. That approval has a number of conditions attached to it (for example rotation arrangements, range of experience), is for a finite period, and if withdrawn disqualifies the post for training purposes which, for most doctors, makes it decidely unattractive. If Trusts wish to keep and attract medical staff they must therefore respond sensitively to Royal College demands.

Following the recommendations of the Calman Report *Hospital Doctors; Training for the Future* the period of specialist training is being reduced from its present average of twelve years to seven years with the inevitable effect that junior doctor training will have to be more intense, efficient and organised. As more junior doctor and consultant time is devoted to the training function so, inevitably, less is available for the service function. On a year-by-year basis, a more intense postgraduate medical education must mean increased training costs, yet there is no suggestion that Postgraduate Deans will provide more funds in their contract with a Trust to offset this cost. Trusts are therefore obliged to manage a widening gap between the demands of their service and training purchasers – both of which are able to employ a contract-based mechanism of accountability to reinforce their demand and reduce the Trusts' room for manoeuvre.

As yet Working Paper 10 consortia and the NHS research funding agencies have not used their contracts to impose stringent conditions upon Trusts. There is every likelihood they will do so, however, as the logic of their newly established contract-based accountability systems works its way through. Working Paper 10 consortia are constituted from groups of Trusts in particular localities which are given the funds previously dispensed by the Regional Health Authorities (RHAs) to purchase non-medical training from colleges of further and higher education (DoH, 1989c). Colleges then sub-contract the experiential training they require from Trusts. Loosely administered at first, this accountability line has become firmer as time has progressed. A similar process of making explicit and answerable an area that was previously hidden and unknown has occurred with the historically dispersed NHS Research and Development (R&D) budget. Its future has been systematically spelt out following the recommendations of the Culyer Report *Supporting Research and Development in the NHS* (Culyer, 1994). Health Authority budgets are to be top-sliced to create a single R&D budget in the NHS. Trusts will have the research element embedded in their existing funding removed and will have to compete for contracts from the central R&D budget if they wish to maintain their research activity (DoH, 1995e: Ch. 2). Again, the effect will be to establish specific accountability measures for a previously unaccountable area of provider activity.

The non-contract-based systems of accountability place different, but no less, demands upon Trusts and, in aggregate, add a further layer of complexity to the bureaucratic web in which they sit. Ultimately, Trusts are accountable to Parliament for meeting their statutory responsibilies and this has been emphasised by the designation of chief executives of Trusts as 'accountable officers' for the stewardship of the public funds under their control (DoH, 1995a: 17). Should Parliament's Public Accounts Committee (PAC) wish to activate this line of accountability whilst investigating a particular probity issue, it therefore has the direct power to do so via the accountable officer. This is of course an unusual occurrence and the routine monitoring of a Trust's financial performance is conducted by an NHSE regional Trust monitoring unit. To carry out its monitoring function a unit requires a Trust to produce an annual business plan, an annual report on the previous year's performance, annual accounts and in-year financial monitoring information (National Health Service Management Executive [NHSME], 1990a: 7). The rules are clear and inflexible: a Trust must make an annual 6 per cent return on the assets transferred to it when it was established (its originating capital debt), break even one year with another, and work within the External Financing Limit (EFL) stipulated by the NHSE (*ibid.*: 16). Furthermore, its financial planning must be carried out according to a strict timetable which results in a business plan being agreed with the regional office by 31 March each year.

This monitoring process is driven by the requirements of the annual Public Expenditure Survey (PES) and is completely at odds with the timetable and requirements of the contracting round driven by a Trust's service purchasing agencies – which also has to be completed by 31 March each year. Normally, an organisation's financial planning is geared to, and sequential to, its business plan. The twin lines of accountability to NHSE regional office and purchasing agencies, however, render this an impossible task for Trusts and means that the two activities must be carried out as two separate and largely unrelated tasks. Should there be a significant problem with either of them then it is likely that a further type of accountability would be activated: the party political line from Trust chairman, through the regional chairman to the Secretary of State. The *Health Service Journal* comments on this mechanism thus:

> A curious paradox has emerged from the NHS reforms: at a time of unprecedented decentralisation in formal organisational terms, the mechanism for political control from the centre [via chairmen] has never been tighter or more effective... Ministers activate this alternative, unofficial management structure – they throw the 'political override' lever – when there are political dangers to be avoided or debts to be repaid. (Health Service Journal, 1993: 17)

For the past ten years this mechanism has been used both as a means of keeping chairmen in touch with the emerging political agenda of the Minister and as an easily activated mechanism for dealing with little local difficulties. Every Trust chairman has to be ready to respond speedily to messages which arrive via this part of the accountability net if they wish to retain their position.

Inside the Trusts

The web of accountability that embraces the so-called 'independent' hospital Trust providers is more sophisticated than any the NHS has experienced before. But sophistication should not be taken to imply coherence. The web is constructed from lines of accountability which carry their messages to separate power centres. Each power centre has its own agenda which may, or may not, be shared with or compatible with those of others. Trusts sit at the centre of the web and are obliged to heed and if necessary reconcile the various messages they receive. Because the buck stops with them they can hardly do otherwise.

At the same time they must continue to carry out their traditional function of rationing the demand for health care, as no Act of Parliament can remove that function from the hands of the medical profession unless the profession so decides. To do so Trusts have been ordained a structure which, except for its upper echelons, is largely unchanged from its pre-1991 hospital manifestation. To what extent does the structural change that has accompanied the establishment of Trusts impact on the ability of the organisation to perform its key rationing function?

As one would expect of institutions described as self-governing within an NHS internal market, Trusts are run by a board of directors with a non-executive chairman and five non-executive directors (appointed by the Secretary of State), a chief executive (appointed by the chairman and non-executive directors) and four other executive directors (appointed by the chief executive and chairman). The appointment procedure ensures that direct central control is retained over the composition of a board. The board is 'responsible for determining the overall policies of the Trust, for monitoring their execution, and for maintaining the Trust's financial viability' (DoH, 1989d: 13).

It is doubtful whether this structural innovation has, of itself, altered the way in which hospitals function. Research into the activities of boards has shown considerable variation in the roles of non-executive directors (Ashburner and Cairncross, 1992; Williamson, 1995), in the way they relate to executive directors (Ferlie and Ashburner, 1993), in the chairman–chief executive relationship and hence in the way boards operate as corporate bodies (Ferlie *et al.*, 1993; Salomans Centre, 1995). In practice, a clear model has yet to emerge. The indications are that the pre-reform officers to the Health Authority continue to carry out their operational tasks as they did before 1990 but are now called executive directors of the Trust. Given this continuity in operational management, the remaining issue is whether boards have a distinctive effect through their probity and strategy functions.

On probity, they have received, and continue to receive, much advice from the Department's Corporate Governance Taskforce and the Audit Commission. In the case of the Taskforce this advice is binding and, in particular, boards are obliged to adopt its codes of conduct and accountability (NHSE, 1994a, b, c). By comparison, the Audit Commission's national reports on corporate governance with their action checklists have the status of good practice so far as boards are concerned (see for example, Audit Commission, 1994a, 1995b) – though there is little doubt that the Commission's statutory auditing of individual Trusts is used as a means for getting its national message across. In practice this means that the secretary and finance director to the Trust have to ensure that the appropriate action is supported and taken by the board or its audit sub-committee as they would have done for the Health Authority.

On strategy, there are no parallel external pressures on boards except for the need to produce one for the regional office's Trust monitoring unit. There is no evidence to suggest that this is then used by the board as a vehicle for driving the organisation along particular paths.

Below board level, Trusts have largely retained the basic format of the structures in place prior to the 1990 legislation, continued the logic of some of the developments already in train and added other organisational features to deal with the new external demands. Following the Griffiths report in 1983 and its optimistic recommendation that general management should help forge the link between clinical and budgetary decision making, there was much debate about the appropriate organisational unit to facilitate this policy. The favoured model which emerged was that of the clinical directorate (BMA Central Consultants and Specialists Committee, 1990; Institute of Health Services Management, 1990; Fitzgerald, 1991a, b). In its pure and rarely realised form, a clinical directorate is a semi-autonomous unit, based on a medical specialty or group of specialties, usually managed by a clinician, to which full budgetary responsibility is devolved and within which clinical and budgetary decision-making are combined.

Supporters of the clinical directorate claim that it will solve the rationing-of-demand problem because, as the District General Manager of Leicester Royal Infirmary put it, using the sanguine phrasing of the Griffiths report, it will ensure:

> that those whose daily decisions in care delivery commit resources must also accept an obligation to be accountable for the effectiveness of their stewardship; that in the context of cash limits, the price of clinical freedom is an acknowledged accountability for resource use, ie clinical management is indistinguishable from resource management. (Barker, 1990: 9)

Behind this confident assertion lies the assumption that it is possible 'to overlay the medical staff organisation on the management hierarchies' in order to achieve 'an organisational bonding' between these hitherto separate entities (Institute of Health Services Management, 1990: 5). Such a reform would require a radical reappraisal of established medical culture and it is scarcely surprising that critics of clinical directorates customarily emphasize the importance of clinical freedom and a return to some form of consensus management (see for example Kennedy, 1990). It is difficult to see how they could argue otherwise.

Within the clinical directorate, it is commonly accepted that its clinical management team (CMT) should be composed of a clinical director, senior nurse manager and business manager; but there is less agreement on the distribution of responsibilities and powers between them and hence 'who is being held accountable for coordinating which aspects of the team's work' (Institute of Health Services Management, 1990: 14). It is also generally, though not invariably, assumed that the clinical director should always be a clinician because, as Connolly observed about the experience of Belfast's Royal Group of Hospitals, it was felt that 'a non-medic would not be able to command respect from senior or junior doctors' (Connolly, 1991: 22). However, given that all consultants in the NHS are created equal, respect may be one thing, authority another. In his account of how Guy's Hospital dealt with the issue of clinical leadership, Chantler observed that 'all consultants in the NHS have equal status and the possibility that any one of them should have authority over others is properly resisted' (Chantler, 1990). His solution was for authority to rest with a group of clinicians with a clinical director taking responsibility for provision of service. Whether a demos of clinicians is a workable proposition is another matter, particularly when decisions have to be made about the allocation of scarce resources between them.

Even if the issue of the degree of authority to be held by the clinical director is resolved, there is the further problem of the motivation of the clinician in management. What has not been addressed is how the clinical directorate can be integrated into the framework of hospital management in a way that provides clinicians with financial and career incentives (Spry, 1990: 10). Within the distinction award system of salary supplements for clinicians, only the lowest category of award includes management responsibility as one of its criteria and it is doubtful whether this is a significant factor in the decision, dominated as it is by clinicians themselves. Trusts do make specific payments to clinical directors for taking on this management role but these are usually too small to act as a serious incentive and are as yet not sufficient to offset the loss of the clinician's private practice which can accompany the assumption of the new responsibilities (British Association of Medical Managers [BAMM] *et al.*, 1993: 30). Some specialties are more prepared to engage in the management process than others. Historically, the diagnostic and support directorates of pharmacy, pathology and radiology have been delegated considerable budgetary and decision-making powers and are more accustomed to managing their own affairs (Grossman, 1990: 14; IHSM, 1990: 6). Nonetheless, the phenomenon of the reluctant clinical director is the pervasive one (see for example, Salter, 1994b: 66–8).

The adoption of the clinical directorate model as a means of engaging clinicians in management has been a slow process. A 1990 survey by the NHSME showed that 40 per cent of hospital units had clinical directorates whilst 80 per cent had at least some clinicians holding budgets (Tomlin, 1990). Three years later, a survey conducted by the British Association of Medical Managers revealed a mixed picture. It found that most providing organisations had a decentralised clinical management structure based on clinical groupings but the proportion of the total unit budget actually devolved to these groupings ranged from under 10 per cent to over 90 per cent with an average of between 50 and 70 per cent (BAMM *et al.*, 1993: 18). It was clear from the latter's research that a 'flattened' clinical management structure was often correctly seen by providers as a necessary condition for Trust status. More than 70 per cent of them had introduced clinical management in 1990 or 1991, usually during the period of preparation for Trust application (*ibid.*: 13).

The introduction of the 1991 reforms accentuated the intensity and specificity of the cost pressures to which clinical directorates have been seen by some as the organisational answer. Trusts and their clinical directorates are obliged to deliver their services to meet the terms of their contracts with Health Authorities and GP Fundholders. As the conditions of the contracts become more precise in terms of quantity, quality and cost (particularly with the advent of The Patient's Charter industry), so Trusts have had to develop the organisational tools to ensure that these conditions are met because the financial penalties for not doing so have become steadily more punitive. The effect of the contractual imperative on the clinical decision-making process has been to try and subordinate clinical freedom to the needs of the Trust: in other words to encroach upon the territory and political autonomy of doctors. In making their clinical decisions hospital doctors are under pressure to reconcile two criteria: (a) what they perceive to be the objective clinical needs of the patient and, (b) the terms of the contract with purchasing agencies. As was discussed earlier, the decision-making associated with the first criterion has always included the means informally to ration demand according to personal predilection. The implication of the second criterion is that this rationing mechanism has to be adapted to deal with the new situation. This is particularly true of those requirements of The Patient's Charter which stipulate the waiting time targets which have to be met by Trusts for out-patient consultations and in-patient treatments (DoH, 1995b: 11–13).

Although there is as yet no firm evidence on how hospital doctors are resolving this conundrum, it is likely that a *de facto* redefinition of clinical freedom will emerge to deal with the demands of the internal market whilst allowing doctors to retain control of their decision-making territory. Despite the profession's suspicion of management, it is the explicit control of resources at the level of the clinical directorate which will give it the bargaining power to resist intrusions. It is already apparent that purchasers have to negotiate with clinicians, as well as with managers, if the contracts they subsequently place with Trusts are to be rooted in the achievable. And on the provider side, it is clear that clinicians are prepared to use their clinical discretion to manipulate their waiting lists in order to satisfy purchaser demands.

Clinician definitions of 'urgent', 'very urgent' and 'emergency' are, up to a point, malleable concepts which can be adjusted to order the flow of patients to satisfy the criteria of both purchaser contracts and clinical assessment. A particular difficulty arises with the 'emergency' category. Where there is contractual flexibility for emergencies only, and none for potential destabilisation in the 'urgent' category of patients, there is an incentive for clinicians to overestimate the 'emergency potential' when selecting patients for investigation and treatment. On the other hand, where there is no contractual flexibility for emergencies a rise in indisputable life-threatening cases can rapidly diminish the amount of decision-making room available to the clinician (Dymond and Lim, 1994: 287). Nonetheless, as the achievement of Patient's Charter targets on waiting times demonstrates, clinicians have been able to adapt their procedures for determining clinical priorities to their Trusts' contractual needs. By so doing they have begun to move the political autonomy of doctors away from a passive reliance on their divine right to allocate resources and towards an active defence of their labour space.

If it is in the combined interest of both the medical profession and service purchasers to develop the clinical directorate as the primary demand-regulating unit, where does this leave the managers as a power group within Trusts? Within the directorates themselves, business managers are the most recent occupational recruits and have to contend with the established professional power of both the senior nurse manager and the clinical director. If the devolution of budgetary and decision-making power to the directorates is real, the role of the business manager is likely to be dependent on how active his/her two colleagues decide to be. If it is not, then he/she is merely the local representative of central management.

The ability of the Trust's central managers to influence what happens inside the clinical directorates, regardless of the formal devolution which has or has not taken place, is constrained by the individual nature of consultants' decision-making; their lack of accountability; the use of historical accident as a guide to operational procedures within directorates; professional divisions and, on occasions, tensions between nurses and doctors; and the absence of any single locus of power complemented by a plethora of informal power networks. It is at the level of the clinical directorate that the long-established culture of the NHS, centred as it is on the principle of medical dominance, is most dense and immutable.

Against this inertia, what levers do managers possess? Regarding clinicians, none that are direct and do not involve argument and persuasion. It is one of the new cardinal freedoms of Trusts that they are able to employ staff on the conditions they consider appropriate and pay them what they want if they so choose (DoH, 1989a: 25; DoH, 1989b). Such a freedom, it was claimed, would give Trusts greater flexibility than their Health Authority predecessors in the way they managed their staffing arrangements. In line with this policy, consultant employment contracts were transferred from RHAs to Trusts and chief executives were made full members of the Advisory Appointments Committees (AACs) which nonetheless continued to be professionally dominated (NHSME, 1991a). Furthermore, it was formally proposed 'to introduce arrangements which will more clearly define the scope and extent of each consultant's duties' (DoH, 1989b: 5). The intention was that each consultant should have a job description which would include the main duties and responsibilities of the post, a sessional (half-day) work programme, participation in medical audit, out-of-hours responsibilities, budgetary and other management responsibities and an annual review (*ibid.*: 6). If implemented and suitably monitored, such a job description was potentially a powerful management tool to restrict medicine's traditional non-accountability and therefore highly provocative to the profession. As yet few Trust managers have chosen to risk the conflict that a thoroughgoing implementation of this proposal would probably produce.

In this they are doing no more than accepting the inherent weakness of their position within the Health Service. Whereas hospital doctors are protected by an array of professional defences which dilute the effectiveness of employment and disciplinary sanctions against them (see Chapter 5), managers are dangerously exposed and maintain their positions on the basis of a one year, renewable contract. Their brief pre-eminence as a result of the post-Griffiths enthusiasm for general management and the change management demands of the internal market policy has been replaced by a marked vulnerability in the party political arena. In April 1994, anxious to offset Labour Party criticism of the burgeoning bureaucracy of the internal market, Virginia Bottomley launched a drive to identify the management costs of Trusts. In its report on the subject, which showed the wide variation in Trusts' management costs, the Audit Commission duly warned that 'To constrain or even reduce management expenditure in the absence of any evidence on what benefits it does or does not achieve, is a dangerous game, however popular it might make the player' (Audit Commission, 1995b: 14). However, as popularity is precisely what the ambitious politician wants, the Audit Commission's caution becomes irrelevant and we find Mrs Bottomley's successor, Steven Dorrell, demanding a 5 per cent across-the-board reduction in Trusts' management spending in 1996 (Warden, 1995a). To use the Minister's own sound bite, there could be no doubt about his preference 'for white coats over grey suits' or for the new political role of managers as scapegoats for NHS problems.

Conclusions

As providers of health care, Trusts are no more immune from the expectations of the population than are the purchasers of health care. Since the foundation of the NHS, a political concordat between the medical profession and the state has ensured that, within hospitals, those expectations are so managed by doctors that they do not totally outstrip the resources available. In exchange for this political service, clinicians received the right to dispose of resources as they sought fit.

Before the introduction of purchasing agencies, hospital doctors had to manage only one type of demand for health care: consumer demand as registered by GP referrals and emergency admissions.

Now there is a second: customer demand as registered through contracts with Health Authorities and GP Fundholders. The two types of demands may or may not coincide. Where they do not, it will ultimately be the task of the clinician to manage both the resulting demand mismatch and the mismatch between the expressed demand and the available supply of health care resources.

At the same time as clinicians have been obliged to respond to new pressures on their rationing function, so Trust organisations as a whole find themselves subject to new and increasingly sophisticated networks of regional and national accountability. On to the existing contracts of the service-purchasing agencies has been grafted a small industry of Patient Charter requirements supported by a highly public monitoring exercise conducted by the Department of Health. Since 1990, contractual arrangements have also become part of Trusts' provision of undergraduate and postgraduate medical education, non-medical education, and research and development – thus introducing precise and measurable forms of accountability into parts of the NHS jungle where finance had previously flowed quiet and undisturbed. Meanwhile the regional bureaucracy, despite its emaciated appearance produced by the unfriendly attentions of successive Secretaries of State, retains a keen interest in maintaining the more traditional lines of control over the hospitals via its Trust monitoring units. Last, but not least, the Minister's personal channel of influence through the regional and Trust chairmen regularly transmits short term political imperatives which vibrate through the accountability networks.

The rise and rise of the accountability web imposes a pluralism of contradictory pressures upon the senior managers of Trusts. Although each individual line of accountability embodies its own logic, the totality of the web does not. Nor is there any reason why it should because the web has been constructed piecemeal in that each accountability component is the formal manifestation of the informal arrangement which preceded it. As these informal arrangements were, in turn, the product of many and varied historical political compromises throughout the long life of the NHS, it would be surprising indeed if the overall effect of the accountability web was anything other than haphazard.

Responsible as they are for the management of the haphazard, Trust managers have to exercise a range of political skills whilst recognising their institutional weakness in the face of the medical profession's long-standing concordat with the state. Externally, they must thread a way through the accountability net, satisfying those that must be satisfied, skirting controversy, negotiating a political fix when it is in the interest of both accountability agency and Trust, and developing obfuscation to the level of an art form. Internally, they must, above all, retain the confidence of their clinicians who, until their rationing function becomes defunct (probably never), will retain the confidence of the politicians.

The organisational means at managers' disposal embody both the aspirations of the 1991 reforms and the reality of medical power. Theoretically Trusts have a range of freedoms not vouchsafed to their Health Authority precessors to employ staff, control their finances and trade with other NHS and private sector organisations as they see fit. In practice, these freedoms are severely constrained, if not nullified, by the unavoidable demands of the accountability web and the need to maintain the confidence of the clinicians. Only the most agile of Trust chief executives will be able to manipulate these constraints to their own advantage.

It was the intention of the reforms that Trust boards should provide the strategic and probity focus for their organisations' operation. While the strategic function is frequently neglected, the significance of the probity function and the role of board non-executives has increased as the accountability pressures have mounted. Below the level of the board, the management task has become more complex as the demands of the accountability web are translated into operational detail. While the continuing development of the clinical directorate, or clinical group, as the primary organisational unit has provided a focus for managerial effort, it remains the territory of the clinician. As such it is the crucible in which the balance is struck between the various demands and the supply of resources. In this context, the role of the clinical director as clinician–manager is pivotal as a way is sought to arbitrate between competing demands, resolve issues of demand–supply mismatch, respect the independence of consultants, and protect the principle of clinical autonomy which legitimises the entire process.

4

Primary Health Care

Introduction

Since the publication of *Promoting Better Health* in 1987, primary health care has steadily moved to the centre of the NHS's political stage. A succession of policy initiatives have combined to expand the responsibilities of primary health care, enhance its status *vis-à-vis* secondary care and increase its share of Health Service funding. In the course of these developments, NHS consumers have been given more primary health care rights with a consequent rise in their expectations regarding the nature and quality of the service they should receive. As with other areas of Health Service activity, the ability of the state to manufacture fresh primary care demand has considerably exceeded the public resources at its disposal to meet that demand.

The political dilemma at the heart of primary care is therefore the customary welfare conundrum of legitimate excess demand over the available supply of state health care. However, what sets primary care apart as a political problem from the rest of the NHS is the historic weakness of its bureaucratic controls. The state has few instruments readily to hand with which to manage this increasingly unruly child.

In exploring the politics at work in primary health care, the chapter begins by examining the way in which the relationship between demand and supply has traditionally been handled in this sector by the medical profession and the NHS bureaucracy. It then assesses the policies initiated by the *Promoting Better Health* and *Working for Patients* White Papers in terms of both intended and actual impact upon this relationship. Third, it reviews the changes that have as a result taken place both within the power structure of primary health care itself and in its interface with the power structures of secondary care.

Traditional demand management

Historically, the untidy organisation of primary health care was the result of the need to accommodate the reality of medical power whilst preserving the semblance of bureaucratic order. This has made life for policy makers extremely difficult. Primary health care services combine Family Health Services (FHS: general practitioners, dentists, pharmacists and opticians) and Community Health Services (CHS: other community health professionals – principally community nurses). Within the Family Health Services category there is the sub-category of General Medical Services (GMS) for the largest medical grouping of general practitioners.

The differences between these categories are more than just terminological. As part of the 1948 settlement with the medical profession on which the foundation of the NHS was contingent, GPs, dentists, pharmacists and opticians retained their status as private practitioners and, unlike their consultant colleagues, refused to become salaried employees of the Health Service. Instead, they received a guaranteed income and capital investment support to be administered through a separate arm of the Ministry of Health. Thus was their clinical, political and economic autonomy assured. In return, they were expected to control the primary health care demands on the state.

Until 1990 when the Family Health Services Authorities (FHSAs) were introduced, the bureaucracy of primary care never pretended to be anything other than a vehicle for passively channeling funds to GPs according to a national formula. Its budget was calculated and administered separately from that of the rest of the NHS: from 1948 to 1974 through executive councils and from 1974–90 by Family Practitioner Committees (FPCs). Their upward lines of accountability ran directly to the Department of Health, by-passing the Regional Health Authorities with their planning and management machinery, and were never politicised to the same degree as those in the acute sector (see Figure 1.1). The Griffiths report and the general management enthusiasms of the 1980s left the FPCs largely unmoved; not surprisingly given that 90 per cent of their budget was demand led, not cash limited, and largely uncontrollable (Audit Commission, 1993: 52). Even the numbers and distribution of GPs were outside the remit of the state bureaucracy, being determined by the professionally dominated Medical Practices Committee.

In contrast to this the Community Health Services have since 1974 sat within the main NHS bureaucracy (prior to that they were within the local authority framework), have generally been located in hospitals and until recently their funding formed part of the overall Hospital and Community Health Service (HCHS) budget. In this position they and their funding were naturally exposed to the political and accountability tides which periodically sweep through the system.

The power and status relationship between the FHS and CHS components of primary health care faithfully reflects the professional hierarchy of the Health Service and reinforces the budgetary advantages and lack of accountability which characterised the FHS. Whilst the Family Health Service is composed primarily of doctors, the Community Health Service is staffed largely by nurses (district nurses, health visitors, community psychiatric nurses, mental handicap nurses, school nurses). It is small wonder, therefore, that the model which came to dominate the FHS/CHS relationship was that of the primary health care team led by the general practitioner. Within this model, community nurses and other non-medical health professionals are 'attached' to a general practice and effectively work within the orbit of GP control. Assiduously propagated by the Acheson and Harding Reports of 1981 (London Health Planning Consortium, 1981; Standing Medical Advisory Committee and Standing Nursing and Midwifery Advisory Committee, 1981), the concept of the primary health care team has never been seriously challenged. As part of the 1986 review of primary health care there was an ill-starred attempt by the Cumberledge Report *Neighbourhood Nursing* to substitute the idea of an alternative nurse-led approach, incorporating nurse practitioners and nurse prescribing, based on sub-divisions of the District Health Authority (DHA) (Department of Health and Social Security [DHSS], 1986a). A year later when *Promoting Better Health* was published, however, the Cumberledge recommendations were brusquely dismissed and the primary health care team approach ('Government policy for many years') reaffirmed (DHSS, 1987a: 40).

General practitioners dominate primary health care for the same reason consultants ultimately determine what happens in hospitals. Both are able to use medical judgements to control the demand from patients and so allow the state to fulfill its obligations to its citizens. However, there is a sense in which the political utility of GPs is greater than that of consultants because they manage the demand on secondary as well as primary health care. It is an unbroken law that except for emergency cases (an increasingly important exception of late) patients can only be seen by an NHS hospital consultant if they have a GP letter of referral. There is no provision in the NHS procedures for patients to have direct access to specialists – that is, to self-refer. As health care systems that allow such direct access generally have higher rates of intervention and higher costs (Carey *et al.*, 1995; Coulter, 1995a), the GP 'gatekeeper' role is of central significance to a state struggling to regulate the effect of rising patient expectations.

Precisely how this critical mechanism works is unknown but its operation is certainly determined by a multiplicity of non-clinical factors. The rate at which GPs refer patients to hospital varies not just within different regions of the country but among practices within defined districts and between GPs in a single practice (Roland *et al.*, 1990: 98). Attempts to explain variation in referral rates as a function of the age of doctors, list sizes, postgraduate qualifications, and practice arrangements have failed, as have analyses based on the standardisation of patient age, sex and case mix (Morrell *et al.*, 1971; Cummins *et al.*, 1981; Armstrong *et al.*, 1988; Wilkin and Smith, 1988). Nor has any relationship been found between high or low referral rates and quality of care and, therefore, as Roland *et al.* observe:

> We do no know whether the patients of doctors with higher referral rates use unnecessary resources and are exposed to unnecessary risks by being referred to hospital. Likewise, it is unclear whether the patients of doctors with low referral rates are being deprived of treatment from which they could benefit. (Roland *et al.*, 1990: 101)

The exercise of clinical judgement remains a sacred mystery and medical professional knowledge an important political resource.

Whilst the GPs' gatekeeper role continued to keep demand for both secondary and primary care within the limits the state's resources could tolerate, then the state had no reason to question the mechanism by which this was achieved. From the state's perspective, that there was no apparent consistency in clinical decision-making was irrelevant so long as patients accepted the legitimacy of their doctors' decisions. But if the state did choose to intervene because of a demand–supply mismatch in health care, the impenetrable nature of clinical discretion made it inevitable that it would still be reliant on the expertise of the medical profession's elite to facilitate this intervention.

Although GPs have always enjoyed the technical political advantage of controlling both the demand for primary health care and access to hospital consultants, the status differential between themselves and consultants has prevented them from realising much political profit from the latter function. Consultants have traditionally occupied a superior position in the medical hierarchy and have used their jurisdiction over waiting lists as the practical means for reinforcing this dominance. Glennerster *et al.* perhaps overstate the case when they describe the GP as 'a supplicant pleading with the consultant on behalf of his/her patient' but there is no doubt that specialists have used their ability to pick and choose patients from a long waiting list as a powerful device to keep their GP colleagues in their place (Glennerster *et al.*, 1994: 5).

The reforms of primary health care

Beginning in 1987, this traditional system of demand management became the subject of a set of reforms with a large and ambitious agenda. Two themes dominate these policies and although a case can be made for their logical coherence it is at best a tenous one. Rather more likely is the view that they simply reflect the continuing tension in the Health Service between rights and resources: a tension which is rarely addressed explicitly. First, there is the emphasis on increasing consumers' primary health care rights. *Promoting Better Health* promised to make primary care services more responsive to the needs of the consumer, raise the standards of care, promote health and prevent illness, and give patients the widest range of choice in obtaining high quality primary care services (DHSS, 1987a: 1–2). To achieve these objectives, GPs were encouraged to take on a range of new health promotion activities (for example, diabetes and asthma clinics), extend their existing vaccination, immunisation and screening programmes (particularly for cervical cancer), and improve the information on their services available to patients. In 1989 *Working for Patients* duly consolidated these rights and *Caring for People* added a complex 'community care' dimension to the health care rights of the elderly, the mentally ill, people with learning disabilities, and the physically disabled (DoH, 1989a, f). (Community care policy is dealt with in Chapter 7.)

The inevitable effect of this policy was to increase consumer expectations and hence intensify the disproportionate demand generated by the primary care sector of the NHS. Between 1978–79 and 1987–88 FHS expenditure had risen more rapidly than expenditure on the rest of the Health Service with the result that the FHS share had increased from 22 per cent to 24 per cent of the total during that period (*ibid.*: 7). Capped at the national level (with the exception of the drugs budget) but open-ended at the local level, the FHS budget was not subject to the same formal constraints as HCHS expenditure and was therefore vulnerable to a swiftly rising demand (Taylor, 1991: 562).

Given this context and the historic weakness of accountability mechanisms in the FHS, the second policy theme has much to do as it addresses the consequent problem of the regulation of primary health care supply in the face of burgeoning, and state legitimated, demand. *Promoting Better Health* flagged up that there was a need 'to improve value for money', to set clearer priorities for the Family Practitioner Services, to redesign the contract with family doctors, and to strengthen the management role of the FPC (created only in 1985), but throughout the document there is the pervasive sense that the state is dependent upon the cooperation and goodwill of its private primary health care providers: general practitioners. Due obeisance is made to the market ideology of the government; for example, 'a greater degree of competition in providing services to patients is the necessary impetus and the combination of a better informed public and a remuneration system geared to consumer demand provides the mechanism' (DHSS, 1987a: 12). But in the absence of a bureaucratic machine to drive policy forward such statements were essentially cosmetic.

At this stage, lacking the appropriate mechanisms for policy implementation, the state was obliged to use persuasion to engage the interest of doctors in its concern with the efficient use of resources. Hence, on referrals, *Promoting Better Health* declared that 'doctors with abnormally high or low rates of referral *will be invited* to take part in an assessment of their approach to help them in making effective use of hospital resources' (*ibid.*: 23, emphasis added). And, on prescribing, it announced that doctors would be provided with information on their prescribing patterns (PACT – Prescribing Analysis and Costs) in the hope that they would both compare their own performance with regional and national averages and engage in voluntary generic prescribing as 'good professional practice' (*ibid.*: 39).

Government, like nature, abhors a vacuum and the search was on for mechanisms which would give substance to the second policy theme of value for money in the delivery of primary health care and its interface with secondary care. Two options were selected, embodying quite different philosophies and structures, which continue to run parallel courses today. They were: (a) the 1990 GP Contract complemented by a re-vamped FPC called the Family Health Services Authority (FHSA) – the managerial solution; and (b) GP Fundholders – the professional solution.

The managerial solution

A joint commentary by the *British Medical Journal* (*BMJ*) and the General Medical Services Committee (GMSC) of the BMA on the 'imposition' of the New GP Contract in April 1990 observed that it had 'resulted in the greatest change in family doctors' terms and conditions for nearly a quarter of a century' (*BMJ* and GMSC, 1992: i). Introduced in the teeth of opposition from the medical profession, the Contract was a clear attempt to provide the new FHSAs with a management tool in their dealings with GPs. It changed the make-up of GPs' incomes by increasing the proportion of doctors' income determined by the numbers of people on their lists ('capitation fees') and by introducing a system of performance-related payments linked to the provision of specific primary care services such as health promotion clinics, immunisation and screening targets, and minor surgery. Management potential the Contract undoubtedly had, but whether the new FHSAs would have the capacity to activate that potential was quite another matter.

Superficially they were different animals from their FPC predecessors. *Working for Patients* and the subsequent NHS and Community Care Act 1990 reduced their Board membership from 30 to 11, introduced general management, and gave them responsibility for ensuring medical audit was carried out by GPs and, last but not least, that prescribing costs were controlled within a fixed FHSA budget administered through a system of indicative prescribing (Department of Health [DoH], 1989a: 56–8). The latter was the most significant departure from previous practice because for the first time a core part of GP expenditure became cash limited – at least so far as the FHSA was concerned. This innovation was a direct response to the increase in NHS drugs expenditure (of which GP prescribing constituted the major share) of four per cent per year above the rate of inflation in the five years up to the publication of the White Paper (*ibid.*: 57). Cash-limited budgets were also introduced for the areas of improvements to GP premises and the staffing of primary care team members directly employed by the practice (DoH, 1989e: 6).

There were those who, from the dizzy heights of the NHS Management Executive, were able to equate organisational relabelling and new paper functions with genuine power shifts at the local level. Thus Andrew Foster, then deputy chief executive of the NHS, wrote in an official National Health Service Management Executive (NHSME) publication that the remarkable degree of autonomy previously enjoyed by independent GP practitioners was now being challenged by the new breed of FHSA general managers (Foster, 1991: 8). He continued:

> the developments of 1990 began to establish the FHS as a managed public service with GPs held responsible for the provision of specified information, and of hours, times and types of service that would have been unthinkable just a few years ago. Existing boundaries between the clinical and the managerial have been tested and have begun to move. (*ibid.*)

Similarly, in the same year the NHSME's *Integrating Primary and Secondary Health Care* claimed that the new GP Contract 'has already shown itself to be a powerful instrument for strategic change in the NHS' and argued that FHSAs should be given greater discretion in managing the Contract to enable them to target efforts and resources on those practices and patients where there is greatest need (NHSME, 1991e: 2–3).

Such statements may be a useful expression of senior management ideology and self-belief, but they bear little relationship to to the difficulties of changing the traditional, and largely passive, administration of the FPCs into a thrusting FHSA management tool for dealing with entrenched medical power. It is instructive to explore what this might mean in order to understand how far, organisationally speaking, the FHSAs had to travel. FHSAs first required a strategic view of what they are trying to achieve to prise them away from their historically reactive stance and to give direction to their management actions. In theory, *Promoting Better Health* gave them such a role through the requirement that FHSAs ensure that the needs of the consumer are duly met. In practice, FHSAs had neither the skilled personnel nor the appropriate strategic information to carry out such a role. Whilst DHAs were able to call upon their public health doctors with their experience of handling morbidity and mortality data to conduct needs identification exercises, FHSAs had no such resource. Furthermore, it has been convincingly argued that the kind of data routinely available to FHSAs (such as morbidity and mortality measures) were not sensitive enough for primary care purposes, were not based on GP catchment areas, and were derived from diagnostic categories which are of limited relevance to primary care provision (Hopton and Dlugolecka, 1995: 1369).

In the event that FHSAs were able to develop a strategic view of primary care provision, they would then have had to deal with the embarassing absence of management controls with which to implement it. In contrast to HCHS funding, the FHS budget is neither calculated nor allocated on the basis of population characteristics (and therefore putative needs) but on the basis of their historic patterns of expenditure which differ considerably from FHSA to FHSA. (One study has shown that the present distribution of primary health care funding is heavily skewed by historical patterns such that the introduction of weighted capitation would produce heavy losses in the south of England and major gains in the north (Centre for Health Economics, 1995).) So the financial logic of FHSA budget-setting did not gel at all with a needs-identification approach. Within the FHS category, 90 per cent of GMS expenditure (payments for services to patients, capitation payments for GP lists, drugs prescribed) was not controlled by the FHSA, nor is it by its Health Authority successor, but was driven by the demand from GPs who do not regard their activities as cash limited (Audit Commission, 1993: 11). Most of the ten per cent balance of GMS expenditure where the FHSA did exercise control and which was cash limited (computers, practice premises, practice staff) was in any case committed in advance (*ibid.*).

The paucity of FHSAs' financial controls was matched by the very limited staffing and information resources available to carry out a positive management function. In 1993 the Audit Commission observed that most staff in FHSAs provided administrative support for General Medical Services – as they had always done. They dealt with GP and practice staff costs, transfered medical records, maintained patient lists, responded to patient complaints and processed applications for activities such as training and new clinics (*ibid.*: 15). As administrative activities, it is not surprising to find that they rarely generated management information in a form useful either to the FHSA or to practices (*ibid.*).

FHSAs were therefore starting from a very low management base, were dealing with independent practitioners unused and unsympathetic to most forms of bureaucratic accountability yet were expected to contribute substantially to the improved efficiency agenda. In the area of prescribing, for example, the government position was that 'the objective of the new arrangements is to place downward pressure on expenditure on drugs in order to eliminate waste and to release resources for other parts of the health service' (DoH, 1989g: 3). The chosen mechanism was indicative prescribing which, building on the PACT system of self-audit by GPs, gave FHSAs the task of monitoring practice drug expenditure against a fixed target on a monthly basis. Regardless of NHSME rhetoric, however, the FHSAs still had to rely on GPs cooperating with the exercise because, ultimately, there was no sanction which could be used against them if they did not.

Lacking both management capacity and management powers, the FHSAs were in no position to use the 1990 Contract as a vehicle for steering primary health care along the path of efficiency and strategic good sense. In the absence of local controls, the Contract simply acted as a set of financial incentives for GPs to expand the range of services they provided according to their individual interests which, in aggregate, produced a random effect. Existing health promotion clinics increased their activity, new ones were established (for example, asthma and diabetes) and GPs paid great attention to reaching their immunisation and cervical cytology targets (Langham *et al.*, 1995; Leese and Bosanquet, 1995). There was wide variation between practices in their take-up of the incentives and, serendipity excepted, little relationship between the provision of new services and the health care needs of the local population. Indeed, the reverse might happen because there was the strong possibility, as Hopton and Dluglecka observe, that by 'encouraging a focus on particular areas of care, national policy may lead to a relative neglect of greater need in areas not linked to financial incentives' (Hopton and Dlugolecka, 1995: 1372).

As the new health promotion and prevention role of the GP became an established part of primary care provision, so it imprinted a permanent mirror image on the expectations of patients. The state had successfully increased the span of the demands placed upon primary care by its citizens without achieving any corresponding impact on the management of the NHS supply. If its managerial solution to the policy problem of the regulation of supply was running into serious difficulties, what of the GP Fundholder option? Would the professional solution be any more successful?

The professional solution

The managerial solution is characterised by a focus on the supply side of the demand–supply mismatch in primary health care and a belief in the efficacy of centrally led managerial action supported by appropriate bureaucratic and contractual mechanisms. In many ways the professional solution is both more radical, more ambitious and, politically, more unstable. Using the system of financial, status and power incentives embodied in the Fundholder scheme, it seeks to delegate to GPs the public responsibility for ensuring a correspondence between supply and demand in both primary *and*, to a degree, secondary care.

Fundholding was introduced on 1 April 1991 under section 14 of the NHS and Community Care Act 1990. From its inception it was designed to embrace the primary–secondary care divide through a judicious blend of providing and purchasing functions incorporated into a single budget. On the provider side, the Fundholder budget included two aspects of GP primary care services: 70 per cent of practice team staff costs, and, most importantly, prescribing (drawn from the FHS budget). On the purchaser side, it included three categories of hospital services: out-patients, a defined group of in-patient and day case treatments and diagnostic tests (drawn from the HCHS budget). Fundholders were also given a fee to cover the management and other costs of participating in the scheme (DoH, 1989a: 49; see also DoH, 1989h). Significantly, each Fundholder's budget, in theory at least, was cash-limited, though Fundholders were allowed virement between the different categories of expenditure. Separate to this budget was the normal GP Contract with the FHSA for the provision of the remaining categories of primary care service.

At the level of Conservative Party ideology, the scheme was justified in terms of enhanced patient choice between competing GPs which, together with general practitioners' new purchasing powers, would act through quasi-market mechanisms to produce improvements in primary and secondary services (DoH, 1989a: 48). More fundamentally, the political logic behind Fundholding was a primary care version of the attempts from the mid-1980s onwards to involve hospital clinicians in management: persuade doctors to take responsibility for working within a fixed budget and leave it up to them and their clinical judgements to reconcile the relationship between the demand and supply of health care. Why did general practitioners agree to accept what some might argue was a poisoned chalice?

It has to be remembered that although general practice has come to be regarded as 'part of the NHS', it is, along with dental practice, opthalmology, and pharmacy, composed of small businesses which contract with the Health Service to provide a primary care service. The financial health of the practice has therefore always been a significant part of GPs' concerns and, as Glennerster *et al.* observe, this may explain why some GPs took to the idea of a competitive market more easily than did NHS managers (Glennerster *et al.*, 1994: 48). To such GPs, Fundholding was simply a step further along a familiar path. It enabled them to improve their businesses with little or no cost to themselves. Hence we find that when asked why they joined the scheme, their stated reasons were to improve the quality of the service they provided, the opportunity to have more services on site, greater freedom of referral, and budgetary freedoms – all sound business motivations (*ibid.*: 46).

Nor would potential Fundholders have been unduly troubled by the accountability mechanisms of the new arrangement since these were virtually non-existent and did not constitute a disincentive. The Fundholder budget was to be determined and allocated by the RHAs (now the regional offices of the NHSE) and monitored by the FHSAs. However, not only was there no contract to underpin the financial relationship between NHS and Fundholder but, as we have already seen, the capacity of the FHSAs to assume any additional management functions was severely limited. Finally, with scant regard for the protection of NHS interests in the allocation of public funds to a private provider, the financial regulations allowed Fundholders to retain any audited underspends on their budgets while overspends were to be met by the funding body (originally the RHA, now the Health Authority) (Audit Commission, 1995c: 19). Heads you win, tails I lose. Health Authorities are 'encouraged to negotiate the return of underspends' but have no powers to claw them back (*ibid.*: 21). The effect of this arrangement was that in 1993–94 three-quarters of Fundholders made a saving (20 per cent of £100 000 or more) and of these about 10 per cent returned part of their underspend (*ibid.*). And in 1994–95 Fundholders overall made £95 million in savings, equivalent to 3.1 per cent of budget; the average practice making a saving of £83 000 (Audit Commission, 1996a: 72). Fundholders are constrained to the extent that savings must be spent in ways 'for the benefit of the patients of the practice' (*ibid.*), but as this can include improvements to the practice premises, and hence the market value of the business property, it does not greatly diminish the incentive to underspend.

There were also status and power incentives. Fundholding held out to general practitioners the possibility that they might reverse, or at least diminish, the historic status and power differences between hospital and general practice that had always divided British medicine (see for example, Honigsbaum, 1979). GPs had never been able to realise the potential advantage embodied in their exclusive power of referral because, for practical and professional reasons, they had needed hospital specialists more than specialists had needed them. Once a GP referral was made, a patient's subsequent progress through the outpatient waiting list, the out-patient treatment, the in- or day-patient waiting list, the in- or day-patient treatment, and discharge back to the GP was wholly controlled by the hospital consultant. GPs might murmur about waiting times or dilatory discharge letters but their professional subordination meant they could not challenge what happened in consultant territory. Consultants meanwhile (of which there is a perennial and, in terms of professional power, useful shortage) have grown adept at manipulating waiting lists to maintain their advantage (see Chapter 3). As *Working for Patients* pointed out, 'hospitals and their consultants need a stronger incentive to look on GPs as people whose confidence they must gain if patients are to be referred to them' (DoH, 1989a: 48). Money is generally a useful incentive and this is precisely what GPs who became Fundholders got.

Not only did the incentives succeed in attracting GPs into the Fundholder scheme, the incentives also became progressively more powerful as their impact became visible to those GPs outside the scheme. Following the entry of the first wave of about 300 practices into the scheme in April 1991, the numbers grew quickly and by April 1996 had reached 2 200, covering about half the population (Audit Commission, 1996a: 8). In April 1993 the British Medical Association (BMA) abandoned its opposition in principle to the scheme and the stage was set for the state to consolidate and expand the power of its chosen professional allies.

The extension of the Fundholder scheme in April 1993 pursued the natural logic of the GP-centred primary health care team and, in so doing, achieved a substantial redistribution of financial power to general practitioners. From within the HCHS budget as a whole, Fundholders were given all the non-acute elements of: the community health services budget (community nursing, paramedical services, specialist nursing); the mental illness budget (day case, outpatients, community); and the learning disability budget (outpatients, community) (Audit Commission, 1995c, Appendix 1). Under the cover of extending an existing policy, the boundaries between primary and secondary care were dramatically redrawn and whole groups of health care professionals (for example, district nurses, health visitors, community psychiatric nurses) transferred to the GP Fundholders' sphere of influence.

At the same time, the criteria for entry into the scheme were progressively relaxed and flexibility introduced by providing GPs with a menu of Fundholding options. In the years following 1991, the minimum list size entry criterion was reduced from 9 000 to 7 000 and then, in 1996, to 5 000. In deciding which version of Fundholding to select, by 1996 GPs could choose from: Standard Fundholding (the original scheme plus the 1993 'community extension' and virtually all elective surgery and outpatient services); Community Fundholding for practices with 3 000 patients or more (community nursing, drugs and practice staff); or practices could combine, pool their management costs and form 'multifunds'. Future directions in Fundholding were flagged up by the establishment in 1995 of 25 'total purchasing' pilot schemes where GPs in a locality would purchase, normally working through a consortium, all hospital and community health care for their patients, including emergency treatment.

The Fundholding policy has clearly succeeded in engaging the professional interest of general practice and to that extent has achieved its first objective. But its utility as an instrument for the rationing of health care, the political *raison d'être* of the policy, as yet remains unproven. A number of key issues are unresolved.

The logic of the professional solution to the supply–demand mismatch in health care assumes that clinical judgement is used to tailor demand so that it fits the available supply. It is a supply-led solution where the doctor is given a fixed budget within which he/she agrees to work. Fundholding GPs now receive two budgets, one of which is fixed (the Fundholding budget) and the other which is open-ended (the GP Contract). While the former pursues the path of the supply-led solution with its built-in rationing assumptions, the latter is demand-led, non-rationing and characterised by task-driven incentives which encourage the expansion of demand in the health promotion areas. Also, there is no simple functional divide between the activities funded by the two budgets: through its prescribing and community health service elements, Fundholding incorporates primary provision as well as its secondary care purchasing role. So in making their clinical decisions, Fundholders are, in theory at least, simultaneously subject to the contradictory impulses of rationing and non-rationing behaviour. What effect has this cocktail of incentives had upon their political utility to the state?

If Fundholding is to work as a rationing agent then it is to be expected that Fundholders will generate less activity, and/or less cost, than non-Fundholders in those areas where they have cash-limited budgets: secondary care referrals and prescribing. On referrals, there is no evidence that the amount, pattern and cost of Fundholder referrals differs from that of non-Fundholders (Coulter and Bradlow, 1993: 436; Dixon and Glennerster, 1995: 727). On prescribing, however, the weight of the research finds that Fundholding reduces costs, or at least the rate of increase in costs, and promotes a greater use of generic prescribing (Coulter, 1995a: 120, 1995b: 236; Dixon and Glennerster, 1995: 727; Whynes *et al.*, 1995). An alternative view based on a longitudinal study is that the differences on prescribing between Fundholders and non-Fundholders have decreased over time – one possible explanation for this being that Fundholders deliberately increased their prescribing costs in their preparatory year (Stewart-Brown *et al.*, 1995).

If the evidence on the rationing abilities of Fundholders is mixed, it has to be noted that this is in the situation where there has been no significant shift in their resource base. Whether this will always be the case is questionable. There is a continuing technical issue around the allocation of Fundholder monies which remains unresolved and has the potential to undermine the legitimacy of the scheme. Funds to a practice are dispensed on the basis of its historic referral, community health service and prescribing patterns, with some negotiable adjustment made in the light of its 'capitation benchmark' (Audit Commission, 1995c: 7). Yet in 1989 *Working for Patients* had proposed that 'each practice's share will be based on the number of patients on its lists, weighted for the same population characteristics as are proposed… for allocation to Districts' (DoH, 1989a: 51): a rational but, as it turned out, politically very difficult policy to implement. The historic and random variations in GP practice activity are such that to re-mould them according to a common formula is to grasp a rather large political nettle and risk alientating GPs. For example, in 1994–95, the amount most Fundholders had to spend per patient varied between £140 and £170, but between the extremes of Fundholders there was a three-fold variation (*ibid.*: 18), and average Fundholder *per capita* budgets also varied between regions. There was no level playing field. In this context it is not entirely surprising that although in the early years of the scheme attempts were made to move to capitation funding, the considerable redistributive implications of such a change produced vigorous resistance from the state's prospective allies, the GPs, and were discontinued.

The consequent absence of a relationship between a population's health care needs and its Fundholders' resources inevitably offends the equity principle at the heart of NHS values. So long as the balance of political costs and benefits serve to keep the issue of the Fundholder allocative mechanism off the public agenda this conflict does not of itself constitute a visible political problem. And this is the case thus far: the development and introduction of a formula funding mechanism is a difficult technical exercise (see for example Sheldon *et al.*, 1994), GP Fundholders can overspend if they run into problems, and the state has every incentive not to alienate them by introducing weighted capitation. However there will come a point in the evolution of the Fundholder policy where its funding mechanism, and hence its rationing principles and abilities, must enter the public realm. The key to this is the relationship between Fundholders and Health Authorities.

With the 1996 NHS Act FHSAs were merged with their neighbouring DHAs to form the new unitary Health Authorities. Among the responsibilities transferred to the Health Authorities was the monitoring of Fundholders. Crucially, the total cost of Fundholding for a given Health Authority became part of that Authority's cash-limited budget for which it was responsible in its corporate contract with the NHSE. If Fundholders overspent, as they were allowed to do, and if this meant that the Health Authority as a whole overspent, this would be regarded as management failure on the part of the Authority and it would be penalised accordingly. There were therefore strong inducements for Health Authorities to try to incorporate Fundholders into a robust set of accountability arrangments.

The attactiveness of such a course of action was reinforced by other pressures. As more GP Fundholders came on stream and assumed their secondary care purchasing role, so funding was transferred to them from Health Authorities. The vagaries of Fundholder budget calculation, however, meant that the amount transferred was generally greater, for the same population, than the amount previously available to the Health Authority under the weighted capitation formula through which it received its funding (Royce, 1995). Health Authorities therefore not only suffered from a shrinking budget, but also a budget that was proportionately and progressively shrinking faster than the population for which it was responsible. At some point the money would run out and the Fundholding allocative mechanism would be exposed to public scrutiny.

Unlike the FHSAs, Health Authorities have at least some management resources with which to construct accountability mechanisms, even though these resources have been reduced by successive anti-management crusades. Yet their ability to mobilise their management potential is severely constrained by the state's commitment to the professional solution to the demand–supply mismatch in primary health care. The professional, GP Fundholder-led solution requires that GPs maintain their long-established NHS status as independent and largely unaccountable practitioners, are given progressively more power, and are trusted to deliver their side of the political bargain. At the same time, the state also requires Health Authorities to deliver a separate management agenda which includes adherence to Patient Charter targets and cash limits.

In such a context, the task of squaring the concept of professional autonomy with accountability for the expenditure of taxpayers' money demands an inventive approach. Official guidance on the issue is naturally bland and evasive. The rhetoric of a primary care-led NHS gives Fundholding the lead and Health Authorities the supporting roles. Thus 'the aim is for decisions about purchasing and providing health care to be taken as close to the patient as possible by GPs working closely with patients through primary health care teams' (NHSE, 1994d: 1). As general practitioners become increasingly important as purchasers, 'Health Authorities need to shift the balance of their activity towards these strategic, monitoring and support [of GPs] roles' (NHSE, 1994e: 2). But when it comes to the 'principles of accountability' which should govern the new arrangements we find that the alchemy of the Fundholder–Health Authority relationship is officially changed and that:

> Health Authorities have statutory responsibility for *leading* the implementation of Government policy at local level. This includes *advising* and *informing* GP fundholders of the wider implications of their purchasing intentions (such as the impact on hospitals or community units or on local strategy) but without second-guessing clinical and management decisions taken by GPs on behalf of their patients (NHSE, 1994g: 3, emphases added).

Fundholders'statutory accountability is still to the NHSE through its regional office but Health Authorities have the day-to-day responsibility for monitoring their performance.

At the rhetorical level, the squaring of the circle between professional autonomy and public accountability is to be achieved through a 'partnership' between GPs and Health Authorities based on mutual respect and rational discussion. However, the experience of locality commissioning, where attempts have been made to involve GPs in the commissioning process using a variety of methods (see for example, Graffy and Williams, 1994), suggests that a reliance on goodwill and good sense is an unrealistic strategy in the political crucible of the local NHS. Glennerster *et al.* have pointed out, apropos locality commissioning, that GPs in a given local area (Fundholders and non-Fundholders) have no shared legal accountability, no shared responsibility for a set budget, and no shared sense that their livelihood is dependent on the viability of 'the locality' (Glennerster *et al.*, 1994: 182). So getting them to cooperate with a Health Authority-led strategy is going to require considerably more than reasoned appeals to their good nature.

In terms of management accountability procedures, GP Fundholders have to submit an annual practice plan to their Health Authority indicating any major shifts in purchasing intentions; submit an annual report to the Health Authority reviewing their performance against the plan; and have regular review meetings with other Fundholders (*ibid.*: 4–5). If they default on any of these procedures, however, Health Authorities have no formal sanctions they can bring to bear. Likewise, the requirements of Fundholders' financial accountability are set out in the *General Practice Fundholders' Manual of Accounts*. According to this document Fundholders should submit annual accounts for independent audit by the Audit Commission, accept monthly monitoring by the Health Authority against their practice plan, secure Health Authority agreement for any proposed use of savings, and deliver their contribution to local efficiency targets (*ibid.*: 7). It is here in the details of financial management that Health Authorities are likely to try and engage Fundholders' interest as they search for a surer footing on the path between professional autonomy and public accountability. If custom and practice can be established in this area, then the political circle may be squared even if the arrangement is not supported by formal sanctions.

The changing power structures

In the long term, the viability of any power structure in the NHS is dependent upon its ability to manage the gap between the rights-driven demand for health care and the publicly funded supply. In recent years, the state's continued sponsorship of primary health care has provided an existing but subordinate power group, the general practitioners, with the opportunity to consolidate a new dominance in the Health Service. To what extent has a redistribution of power taken place and how permanent is it likely to prove?

As the largest portion of primary care, General Medical Services has never experienced any serious rivalry from the other constituent parts of pharmacy, opthalmology and dentistry. Pharmacy was never a political issue because pharmacists do not have any effect on the demand for pharmaceuticals but simply act to supply the demand generated by GP-prescribing. Opticians were eliminated as a factor in primary care by the removal of their monopoly over the supply of spectacles in 1984 and the ending of the NHS provision of spectacles in 1986. And NHS dental treatment has never been free at the point of delivery and there has always been a price mechanism (dental fees) to regulate the relationship between supply and demand.

In terms of rhetoric, money and services, GPs enjoy an enhanced position. The continued shift towards 'a primary care-led NHS' is driven by the financial muscle of GP Fundholders which is redefining the traditional relationship between primary and secondary care. Through their role as purchasers of secondary care, Fundholders are seeking to challenge the entrenched decision making power of hospital consultants and, over time, the status assumptions which have governed much of the GP–consultant relationship. Their control of an increasing proportion of hospital funding means that they are able to use contractual definitions of quality and standards to insist that certain targets are met regarding, for example, waiting times for patient appointments, standards of care, and the speed at which discharge letters are received (Glennerster *et al.*, 1994: 68–70). Some parts of the hospital service, and some consultants, are more responsive than others to the potential loss of GP Fundholder income and hospital managers may act as a conduit for Fundholder pressure where a consultant either does not perceive the pressure or regards it as illegitimate. The most dramatic improvements have been reported in pathology where the service is specific, technical and least open to the exercise of clinical discretion. At the same time, some GPs have begun to provide, or through their purchasing function have chosen to transfer from hospital to the community, services previously seen as the exclusive property of secondary care: for example, minor surgery, chronic disease management, near patient diagnostic testing, outreach hospital clinics, and hospital at home schemes.

The advantage now enjoyed by GPs in their relationship with secondary care is matched by the consolidation of their position within primary care itself. The 1990 Contract gave them the lead in the field of health promotion and, in practical terms, quietly allowed them to undermine the traditional role of the public health doctors as promoters of health and preventors of disease (Hannay, 1993). With the 1993 'community extension' to Fundholding, much of the responsibility and budget for the hospital-controlled Community Health Services was transferred to GP Fundholders. Before this change, GPs had direct influence only over those professionals they employed – principally practice nurses which, from the late 1980s onwards, had experienced a large, centrally supported expansion programme. Control of the CHS budget now allows Fundholders to integrate into the primary health care team on their own terms a whole range of community health professionals (for example, district nurses, health visitors, community psychiatric nurses) whose professional subordination is now explicit. (Generally speaking, these professionals are employed by Community Trusts and supplied under contract with the Fundholders.)

If the political gains of general practitioners are to be turned to their permanent advantage, the state must be convinced that its commitment to a primary care-led NHS will produce a lasting solution to the demand–supply mismatch in health care. One of its more or less explicit assumptions, vigorously encouraged by the health promotion lobby, is that investment in primary care can produce a reduced demand for hospital care either through the early diagnosis of a condition or through the substitution of treatment. The evidence suggests that this assumption is false. Rink *et al.* found that the introduction of near patient diagnostic testing by twelve practices increased the demand for testing but did not reduce the demand for specialist care (Rink *et al.*, 1993). Similarly, the introduction of a minor surgery service into practices encouraged more people to come forward for treatment who would not otherwise have done so and had no impact on the demand for hospital services (Lowy *et al.*, 1993). On the broader national canvas, the Audit Commission found no substitution effect in the variations of expenditure by the community health service, hospitals, FHSAs and social services. Indeed, it reported that the reverse happens: 'the more a district spends on hospitals, the more it is likely to spend on community health services' (Audit Commission, 1992a: 12). More primary care supply does not mean less secondary care demand.

In 1948 the Labour government assumed that there was a finite amount of ill-health in the population and that the demands on the NHS would reduce as the health of the population improved. However, this did not happen because the demand for health care is driven at least as much by individuals' expectations of their rights in a free Health Service, as by their objective medical condition. Nothing has changed. As the range and supply of NHS services in primary care is expanded, so new expectations and demand are created, existing ones are maintained, and so the supply is always insufficient. As the public opposition to the closure of any hospital vividly demonstrates, the provision of more sophisticated primary care does not act as a substitute in the popular imagination for the continued appeal of specialist acute care. Nor is the GP's role as gatekeeper to secondary care immune to the pressure from patients for referral for specialist opinions (Armstrong *et al.*, 1991).

Against this it can be argued that the key shift to a cash-limited budget for which the general practitioner is explicitly and directly accountable has yet to be achieved. Furthermore, that until the sieve-like quality of the present budgetary and accountability arrangements in Fundholding and primary care are rendered more watertight, there are no serious incentives for GPs to engage in more rigorous rationing behaviour. Until they do, and until it is then possible to evaluate their utility to the state as rationing agents, their future power position in the NHS must remain an open question.

Conclusions

For most of its history, the major component of primary health care, the Family Health Service, escaped the attentions of policy makers bent on making more efficient use of the NHS's finite resources. Its bureaucracy was underdeveloped and administrative in character, it depended on providers who were professionally and legally independent and highly resistant to any central direction, and it was exempt from cash limits. However, provided the FHS delivered the political service of reconciling the primary health care demands of the population with the limits of the public purse there was no reason why the state should seek to intervene. Hence it was only in the mid-1980s when the rise in the uncapped FHS expenditure was proportionately greater than that of the NHS as a whole that the warning signs were triggered and the state was obliged to act.

Given the nature of the welfare state hegemony, it was inevitable that the ensuing policies on primary care would emphasise patient rights as much as resource constraints. This *Promoting Better Health* duly did, thus giving the spiral of health care demand an extra push before dealing with the issue of the correspondence between that demand and the available supply. Patients were promised a range of new services, particularly in the areas of health promotion and prevention.

To deal with the correspondence issue, the state proposed two solutions. First, the managerial solution which placed its faith in the metamorphosis of the largely passive administrative structure of the FPC into a more forceful system of accountability capable of delivering both national and local priorities. A central component of this revamped bureaucracy was to be the new 1990 GP Contract driven by a complex system of financial incentives. In the event, it was the general practitioners who found it easier to manipulate the conditions of the new Contract than did the managerially inexperienced FHSAs. Despite increased downward pressure on costs from the NHSE and the imposition of cash limits in selected categories of expenditure such as prescribing, the FHSAs were never able to achieve the qualitative bureaucratic leap forward required of them. Instead, GPs have retained their legal and professional independence and have yet to find themselves subject to the web of accountability systems which envelop the acute sector.

Second, the state advanced the policy of GP Fundholding: the professional solution. Whereas the managerial option is a top-down rationing policy, driven by the local arm of the NHS bureaucracy and focusing on primary care, Fundholding is altogether more ambitious. It seeks to delegate to GPs the responsibility for rationing primary and secondary care through a system of financial and status incentives over which the state has only the flimsiest of controls. Fundholders are asked to work within a fixed budget for the secondary services they purchase and the drugs they prescribe and in return have been given greater financial autonomy and the opportunity to improve their professional status. Armed with their considerable purchasing power – which now includes the Community Health Services budget – Fundholders are in a position to pressurise their consultant colleagues in a way which their subordinate status within the medical profession had previously rendered unthinkable. How far such financial realpolitik will result in a reordering of the traditional medical, and hence NHS, status hierarchy will depend on the staying power of GPs as rationing agents, their unity as a professional group, and the nature of the compromise they must ultimately strike with the requirements of public accountability.

Thus far the state has deliberately done nothing that might undermine the attractiveness to GPs of the professional solution to the demand–supply dilemma in primary care. In particular, the state has carefully avoided insisting that GP Fundholders accept the kind of accountability mechanisms at work in the rest of the NHS. The principle of the cash-limited budget on which any rationing exercise depends has scarcely been enforced: Fundholders can keep their underspends and are not held responsible for their overspends. With the merger of the FHSAs and DHAs to form the new Health Authorities in 1996, however, a new factor has entered the situation. Although Fundholder budget setting and allocation remains the responsibility of the NHSE's regional office, the aggregate Fundholder budget for a given Health Authority now forms an integral part of that Authority's overall allocation and, as such, is subject to the normal requirement to balance the books or suffer the consequences. As a result Health Authorities, lacking any formal authority to ensure Fundholder compliance with the normal tenets of NHS financial management, are energetically seeking to develop informal methods for ensuring Fundholder accountability. It is in the nature of the balance struck between the professional autonomy of general practitioners, on the one hand, and the necessary management of public funds, on the other, that the political future of primary care must lie.

5

Medicine

Introduction

The foundation of the National Health Service in 1948 was contingent upon an appropriate concordat being struck to resolve the tensions between medicine and the state. In essence, the political solution was the time honoured one of mutual advantage: the medical profession gained money, status and the power to protect and regulate its privileges; the state gained a health care system to protect and regulate its populace. Convenient to both sides, the concordat has remained substantially unchanged over the last five decades. But in recent years a variety of pressures have combined to render the arrangement at best anachronistic and at worst obselete.

While a redefinition of the concordat may be potentially advantageous to both medicine and the state, the complexity of the long standing agreement, coupled with the tangled lines of power and influence which link the two sides, mean that negotiations are bound to be lengthy and arduous. In analysing the politics of the concordat, this chapter begins by identifying the basis of medical power, the nature of the state's interest in the profession and the pressures for change. Second, it unravels the web of tensions within the medical profession's mechanisms of self-regulation which renders its internal management of change less than straightforward. Finally, it discusses the likelihood of a new concordat emerging and the form it may take.

Professional power and the pressures for change

The power of the medical profession is based on its unique access to, and control of, a body of knowledge which is highly valued by both society and state. Formal recognition by the state of the profession's control of medical knowledge came with the passing of the 1858 Medical Act and the establishment of the General Medical Council (GMC). This legislation granted the profession exclusive rights to, and hence a legal monopoly over, the practice of healing. At the same time, the Act resolved a number of existing tensions within medicine and thereby, as Porter remarks, 'proved an ingenious compromise, placating the reformers, protecting the profession and ensuring that in the resultant readjustment of territorial boundaries, none of the regular profession came out as losers' (Porter, 1987: 51). But the most important political principle established by the Act was that of professional self-regulation.

With the creation of the GMC, the occupation of medicine was given the right to determine its own standards of practice and regulate its membership through the GMC's registration and disciplinary procedures. When coupled with the profession's existing rights to select, train, recruit, and promote its membership, this formal recognition by the state of the right to self-regulation consolidated for medicine a position of formidable occupational power. There are two strands to the ideological justification for this unusual arrangment, both rooted in the profession's control of medical knowledge. First, in the words of the Committee of Inquiry into the Regulation of the Medical Profession (chaired by Sir Alec Merrison), self-regulation can be seen 'as a contract between the public and the profession, by which the public go to the profession for medical treatment because the profession has made sure it will provide satisfactory treatment' (Merrison Report, 1975: 3). Second, again in the words of the Merrison Report, self-regulation is necessary because 'it is the essence of a professional skill that it deals with matters unfamiliar to the layman, and it follows that only those in the profession are in a position to judge many of the matters of standards of professional conduct which will be involved' (*ibid.*). So not only is self-regulation in the public interest, runs the argument, but it is also a consequence of the nature of medical knowledge *per se*. At the level of the individual practitioner, the two strands combine to produce the principle of clinical autonomy: that it is the doctor's right to use his unique access to medical knowledge to make his clinical judgments purely in the patient's interest uninfluenced by anything other than the opinion of his peers.

In ceding the principle of self-regulation, the state bestowed upon the medical profession exceptional political power. In return it received a formal guarantee that the service delivered by the profession would be of a satisfactory standard. Also, the state was reassured that the coterie of medical elites to which the 1858 Act gave legitimacy would provide stability in a key area of the state's responsibility and would act on the state's behalf to deal adequately with the political pressures which that responsibility generated.

The move from a mid-nineteenth century bargain of limited, though significant, scope to a mid-twentieth century concordat of considerable complexity between medicine and the state was made necessary by the state's expansion of the social rights embodied in the concept of British citizenship. Following the recommendations of the Beveridge Report, the welfare legislation of the 1945–50 Labour government gave new rights to citizens which, in turn, created new political expectations and, in the context of an electoral democracy and universal suffrage, fresh and unavoidable demands upon the state. In particular, the creation of the NHS in 1948 promised universal health care for all of the population, free at the point of delivery, from the cradle to the grave. In this situation, renegotiation of the state's historic relationship with medicine was an urgent political imperative: only the medical profession could act on behalf of the state to control the demand for health care which the state's own actions had so assiduously cultivated. Now that price no longer constrained that demand, the medical profession itself was the only alternative mechanism.

In return for the use of its monopoly of the practice of healing as a means for implementing the new policy and regulating the impact of the new rights, medicine requested and obtained three things in exchange: reaffirmation of its monopoly position and its right to self-regulation, economic security, and dominance over the allocation of NHS resources. Having manoeuvred itself into a position where it was dependent upon the medical profession to deliver its policy, the state was in no position to argue and the concordat was born.

The 1948 concordat was a product of the state's self-imposed need to redefine its relationship with medicine and the balance of power within the concordat reflected that essential weakness on the part of the state. The extent to which medicine exploited this weakness to shift the balance in its favour can be understood in terms of the profession's enhanced autonomy (see Chapter 3). As a result of the 1858 Act it already had clinical autonomy (the right to regulate its own affairs) and the new arrangement gave it economic and political autonomy as well. Economically, doctors were assured of employment either as salaried employees of the NHS (hospital doctors) or as private practitioners (GPs, dentists, opticians, pharmacists) with guaranteed arrangments for the continuation of their private practice. Politically, they were given control of the disposal of NHS resources through their unquestioned right to make their clinical decisions as they saw fit. Their only accountability was to their professional peers. Clinical autonomy thus led unerringly to political autonomy. The state could still decide on the total budget of the NHS but the medical profession would determine how it was spent.

Although the clinical, economic and political autonomy of medicine had undoubtedly been increased, this had been achieved through the exercise of what was essentially negative or blocking power. The historic divisions between medicine's controlling elite institutions (the Royal Colleges, Universities, GMC and the British Medical Association (BMA)) and the rigid status differences between hospital consultants and GPs does not make the profession an effective fighting force when on the offensive. But in defence these divisions coalesce into barricades. So long as the state needed medicine more than medicine needed the state that blocking power would remain an effective political weapon and would maintain the concordat regardless. But if the balance of dependency became uncertain, a more complex political relationship would have to emerge if the concordat was to remain viable.

Over recent years a number of factors have combined to challenge the power of the medical profession and destabilize the concordat. At the most basic level, there has been a questioning of the profession's unique access to medical knowledge in terms of both the principle and the practice of that access. Not only has technology made this knowledge more available to non-doctors but patients today are much more likely to challenge clinical decisions – as is indicated by the steady increase in complaints about medical care (Elston, 1991: 79). As an editorial in the *British Medical Journal* observed, 'the rise of the sophisticated consumer' is a driving force for change in medical practice:

> No longer patient, these sophisticated consumers and their agents are challenging the unique authority of doctors and insisting on a greater role in clinical decision making. Patients cannot be treated as passive fodder for medical practice. Increasingly patients are as educated as their doctors... The doctor–patient relationship, which many see as being at the heart of medicine, will change fundamentally. (Morrison and Smith. 1994: 1099)

The same point was strongly emphasised by Sir Maurice Shock when, in November 1994, he opened the first 'summit' meeting of the profession since 1961: 'instead of the rights of man we have the rights of the consumer, the social contract has given way to the sales contract, and, above all, the electorate has been fed with political promises... about rising standards of living and levels of public service'. He warned the profession,' everything is different except the way you organise yourselves. (Smith, 1994: 1248)

Those who argue in favour of what has been called 'the deprofessionalisation thesis' claim that the change in patient attitudes is symptomatic of a general decline in the cultural authority and legitimacy of the medical profession (Haug, 1973, 1988; Starr, 1982). Certainly there can be little doubt that the rise of the neo-liberal New Right in British politics has provided ideological legitimacy for consumer assertiveness in the health care arena through its emphasis on consumer power, competition, and more easily available information on medical outcomes (see for example Redwood, 1988; Green *et al.*, 1990; Gladstone, 1992). At the same time, and paradoxically, there has been the rise of state-sponsored (rather than market-driven) consumer rights in the form of the continually evolving requirements of The Patient's Charter with its supporting bureaucracy of national monitoring and reporting systems. If patients' rights are not fulfilled then logic dictates that the state should ensure that there are the means for registering a complaint: hence the review of NHS complaints procedures by the Wilson Committee and its report *Being Heard* (DoH, 1994a). This was swiftly followed by *Acting on Complaints* which provides central guidance to all organisational units of the NHS on the establishment of new complaints procedures which are to have statutory backing (National Health Service Executive [NHSE], 1995b). And so the industry grows.

If the legitimacy of the profession's clinical decision-making is questioned by the consumers of medical care (and with the active connivance of the state), it follows that the effectiveness of its clinical autonomy is also reduced because the profession is no longer able to dictate the terms on which it interacts with this part of its environment. Most importantly from the state's point of view, any reduction in the perceived legitimacy of the profession to determine what is, and what is not, appropriate medical care must inhibit its ability to regulate the public's demands on the NHS. For if the public no longer automatically accepts the authority of doctors' definition of medical need, the political value of the profession and its contribution to the concordat is correspondingly diminished.

If the clinical autonomy of doctors is under challenge from consumers, their political autonomy within the NHS is under siege from both managers and policy-makers. The first serious attempt to limit this autonomy came with the report of the inquiry into the management of the NHS, chaired by Sir Roy Griffiths, in 1983. The Griffiths Report argued that a general management function should be introduced into the NHS and coupled with an increased role for clinicians in the active management of their budgets. The intention was to make clinicians more accountable. However, although the creation of a linkage between clinical decisions and finite resources may constrain the exercise of clinical autonomy, it will have no impact on the political autonomy of doctors if, in line with the terms of the concordat, they remain accountable solely to their patients and their profession. They will simply make their management decisions in the light of their professional needs – which may, or may not, coincide with the needs of their host organisation. Their political autonomy will be threatened only if their accountability is extended to include a dimension of corporate responsibility.

Despite the rhetoric of general management it seems unlikely that the post-Griffiths attempts to reduce the political autonomy of doctors, either by drawing them into the management process or by making them directly accountable to their host organisation, had much significant impact (see Chapter 3). What these policy initiatives did demonstrate was the sheer inertia of the system and the difficulty of shifting an established power interest embedded at all levels of the NHS. Because the NHS had been constructed around the reality of medical power this conclusion was, with hindsight, the predictable one. Ensconced as it was within the labyrinthine bureaucracy of the NHS, up to the late 1980s medicine could use its traditional blocking power to obstruct changes which it viewed as detrimental to the profession (Thompson, 1987). Its economic autonomy, after all, remained unquestioned and there had never been any suggestion that economic sanctions should be used against the profession and in support of the general management policy.

But with the 1989 NHS Review and the 1990 NHS and Community Care Act a fresh political agenda emerged posing quite different questions for the medical profession. The objective of the reforms was to fragment and decentralise the established bureaucracy of the NHS through the introduction of an internal market based upon purchaser agencies and provider Trusts. Trusts were to have a range of powers and freedoms not available to Health Authorities and, in particular, 'should be free to employ whatever and however many staff they consider necessary' depending upon their service needs (Department of Health [DoH], 1989b: 25). As their service needs would in turn depend upon their performance in the market and their ability to attract contracts from the purchasing agencies of Health Authorities and GP Fundholders, so also would their requirements for medical staff. It has taken some time for the logic of this policy and its implications for the medical profession to sink in.

The primary effect is that there is pressure for the clinical, political and economic autonomy of clinicians to become contingent upon the corporate interest and performance of their employing Trust. In practical terms this means there is pressure for clinical decisions to be related to the contractual commitments of the Trust, for clinical activities to be integrated with its management structure and for clinicians' employment contracts and conditions of service to be adjusted to suit the Trust's corporate needs. However, although the formal logic of the situation dictates that the Trust's corporate needs be given priority over professional concerns, the counter logic of the NHS's traditional, and still dominant, political culture suggests that it is unwise to make this argument explicit. Thus, at one level, Roy Lilley, then chairman of Homewood Trust, was simply stating the formal logical position when he listed three priorities for medical staff:

> The first duty is a loyalty to the organisation they work in. The second duty of doctors is to themselves. They must get themselves organised and properly trained. Only when doctors work as part of a team, agree to be properly qualified, tested and brought up to date, can they discharge their third responsibility – their duty to patients. (Pallot, 1994: 7)

But at another level he was challenging the concepts of medical autonomy embodied in the concordat.

In the case of hospital doctors, the effect of the 1991 reforms has been to expose them to pressures from which the traditional NHS bureaucracy had protected them. Doctors in general practice are in a different position (see Chapter 4). As GP Fundholders or members of GP purchasing consortia, they have had to act both as purchasers of secondary care (with a fixed budget) and providers of primary care (with an open-ended or indicative budget). In order to implement these arrangements while continuing to carry out their function of regulating the demand for health care, GPs have had to take on an enhanced management role. Unlike hospital doctors, they have always had to manage their own practices but their new purchasing function, coupled with an expansion of the range of services they provide (for example minor surgery), substantially increased the complexity of their management tasks.

Assuming that they carry out these tasks efficiently, GPs will have improved the terms on which they relate to their environment and thereby increased their political autonomy. However, the fact that at least part of their work, and probably in the future all of it, is conducted within a fixed budget means that their economic autonomy will depend on (a) their skill in managing the resources available to them and (b) the extent to which patients accept the legitimacy of their clinical decisions (their clinical autonomy) and hence the right and ability of GPs to ration the demand on their budgets.

Finally there are the pressures arising from Britain's membership of the European Union and the drive to 'harmonize' the training and accreditation of doctors throughout Europe. It is an interesting tribute to the British medical profession's resistance to change that although the 1975 European Community Directive governing the mutual recognition of qualifications came into force in Britain in 1977, it was only following the European Commission's threat of infraction procedings in 1992 that the Calman Inquiry into the post-graduate training of hospital doctors was established. As we shall see shortly, the implications of the consequent report for the power structure of British medicine are considerable. At the same time, rapid developments in medical technology have placed the existing system of continuing medical education (CME) under significant pressure to provide the profession with the appropriate updating of its skills and knowledge base.

From the state's point of view, the political significance of medicine is that it can regulate the demands from the citizenry. The constant increase in social rights resulting from the competition between the political parties to create fresh categories of citizens deserving of state support has created an upward spiral of expectations that would have placed the concordat under strain in any event. When combined with the pressures on the medical profession resulting from changing consumer views, radical policy initiatives and a reluctant recognition of the requirements of European membership, a revision of the concordat is now inevitable. But for the concordat to be redefined, medicine's internal power structure of self-regulation will first have to be reviewed, as it is this which determines the profession's capacity to respond to the pressures for change.

Over the last century, the self-regulating mechanisms of the medical profession have undergone only incremental change. Situated as they are in the power orbits of the universities, Royal Colleges, GMC, BMA, and a network of medicine-dominated government committees, these mechanisms have thus far been protected by the system of medical elites established by the 1858 Medical Act and confirmed by the 1948 concordat. Historical continuity in a rapidly changing world is not necessarily a bad thing, but in the case of medicine the original faults inherent in a fragmented system of self-regulation have been preserved almost intact. This is of interest for political as well as archeological reasons. It is a raw demonstration of the power of an ascendent profession, but a profession with no experience of the internal management of change.

The state allows the medical profession to regulate itself on condition that this arrangement best serves the interests of the public. In policing itself in order to achieve this purpose and so protect the concordat, the profession must concern itself with all aspects of its members' activities likely to affect the service provided to the populace. These activities, and hence the regulating mechanisms, can be categorised in terms of training and accreditation (entry into the profession), career structure (progress through it), and maintenance of professional standards (possible exit). The pressures for change have been, and are, acting on the three areas of self-regulation in different ways. Each is analysed in terms of the political problem facing the medical profession, its likely response and the internal redistribution of elite power to which this may give rise.

Training and accreditation

There is no single system of medical training but rather a loose collection of professionally dominated institutions bound together by informal understandings and procedures. These arrangements are characterised by diverse lines of accountability paralleled by at best imprecise, and at worst unknown, lines of funding. Such changes as have been introduced over the past century have necessarily been the result of lengthy negotiations between numerous medical power centres with the state acting as bemused banker and onlooker. Although there have always been tensions within the organisation of the NHS between training and service needs, in the past these differences have never challenged the ability of the medical profession to regulate its own training affairs. But with Trusts now under a new imperative to respond to the demands of their purchasing agencies in a cost-effective manner, any factor which inhibits that response or reduces its efficiency may be seen as acting against the corporate interests of the Trust.

In analysing how medical training and accreditation is likely to deal with this new situation, this chapter considers, first, undergraduate training and, second, postgraduate training and continuing medical education (CME).

Undergraduate medical education (see Figure 3.1)

Universities accredit undergraduate medical education and their medical schools take responsibility for its delivery on a day to day basis. However, in doing so they act within two constraints. The annual total of medical students entering training (about 4,500 in 1993) is determined by DoH committees and the distribution of places and money by the Higher Education Funding Councils (HEFCs) of England, Wales and Scotland which are accountable to the Department for Education and Employment (DFEE). So any change in the overall shape of undergraduate medical training has to be implemented through this bureaucratic net. At this point we turn to the Education Committee of the GMC which, interestingly, has precisely that general responsibility for medical education. According to Section 5 of the Medical Act 1983 the Education Committee 'shall have the general function of promoting high standards of medical education and coordinating all stages of medical education' by determining the knowledge and skills, standard of proficiency, and patterns of clinical experience offered by medical schools (Department of Health and Social Security [DHSS], 1983b, Section 5, paras 1 and 2). Unfortunately there is no formal link between the responsibilities of the GMC for medical education and the funding power of the bureaucratic net of the DoH, DFEE and HEFCs. The GMC has only the power of persuasion exercised through 'the issue of Recommendations..., the convening of conferences and the provision of general advice and encouragement about standards at the national level' (GMC, Education Committee, 1987: 20). Its claim that the Education Committee's 'responsibility for standards is linked to provisional and full registration' has to be seen as disingenuous (*ibid.*): there is no evidence of the registration power being used to insist that certain training standards are met. In practice, the Committee's powers are limited to a medical school visit and report for, as a *British Medical Journal* editorial observed whilst commenting on the GMC's difficulties in implementing curriculum reforms, its 'only [other] sanction is like a nuclear deterrent – it can close a medical school, but it is never going to do that' (*British Medical Journal*, 1994: 361).

Even if the GMC did have access to the levers of funding in undergraduate medical education, its position would be scarcely improved, as these levers have never been used as instruments of accountability. Hence, very little data exists on the costs of medical students because such data has never been needed (Hann, 1993). In 1992, the Medical Manpower Standing Advisory Committee (MMSAC) estimated the total cost of undergraduate training at £180 000 per student but was able to further divide this only into two figures: £75 000 through the HEFCs for medical school funding and £105 000 through the Service Increment for Teaching and Research (SIFTR) for the cost to the NHS of providing the necessary teaching and research support in hospitals (MMSAC: 1992: 67). So far as the Universities–NHS funding relationship was concerned, this imprecise state of affairs had been expressly justified by the principle of 'uncosted mutual assistance' contained in the DHSS guidance (HM[73]2) drawn up jointly with the University Grants Committee (UGC) in 1973 and never challenged or amended since (National Health Service Management Executive [NHSME], 1991f: 29–30). Vagueness was legitimate because non-accountability was the norm.

The separation of funding mechanisms from the GMC's statutory responsibilities for the quality of medical undergraduate training has produced a fairly nominal system of professional self-regulation, with predictable results. For example, research undertaken in the context of the GMC guidelines *Recommendations on General Clinical Training* has revealed particular problems in the pre-registration year following undergraduate training. It shows pre-registration house officers (PRHOs) in hospitals experiencing inadequate induction and spending much of their time in inappropriate tasks, either beyond or below their competence, with inadequate supervision by consultants (Dowling and Barrett, 1992, quoted by Lowry, 1993: 60–3). Commenting on the same guidelines from the consultants' perspective, Wilson points out that they receive no training in educational methods, that dedicated time for training is difficult to find, and that 'the GMC's appeal for the goodwill of consultants to underwrite the improvements in house officer training... comes at a time when this commodity is losing ground from competing demands' (Wilson, 1993: 195). Even the numbers are wrong. A Minister for Health, Brian Mawhinney, chose to highlight what he called 'the major distributional anomalies in PRHO posts' (Mawhinney, 1994).

The inability of the GMC to regulate a training system over which it has little or no practical control has produced an accountability vacuum which, under external pressures for change and in the absence of any central policy initiative, is likely to be filled by the use by individual institutions of detailed contracts as the accountability mechanism. Leicester University's medical school, for example, has chosen to allocate its SIFTR funding to local hospitals for the service component of its students' training on the basis of what teaching the students say they have had, not on what the hospitals claim to have provided. Because the allocations are made to individual hospital departments, this has made these departments considerably more 'responsive' to the University's training requirements (Lowry, 1993: 56). Similarly, the University of London has issued guidelines on what is acceptable in a house officer's post and warned that jobs failing to come up to standard would not be recognised by the University (Richards, 1992). On the other side of the coin, the demands of an increasingly cost-conscious NHS mean that Trusts providing a training context for undergraduates now have a clear incentive to ask whether the income they receive from the SIFTR contract covers the true cost of the training service provided. Historically, this cost, which includes items such as early patient admission, the use of experimental procedures for learning purposes and consultant time, has never been calculated but now, under the pressures of the contract-driven NHS, may well have to be.

For the future, two factors are likely to encourage the development of accountability mechanisms in undergraduate medical training, though in neither case will it enhance the regulatory role of the GMC. First, the implementation of the recommendation of the Culyer Report on research and development that the 'R' component of the SIFTR allocation should be transferred to a distinct, and quite separate, research funding stream, means that medical schools are doubly anxious to get value for the reduced funds available for their students' hospital-based training (Culyer, 1994). Second, the HEFCs will shortly introduce a mechanism which will both monitor the quality of the teaching provided in University departments and adjust the allocation of funds accordingly. As part of this exercise, medical schools will become more accountable to the HEFCs. How the medical profession will be integrated into this process, apart from on an informal and *ad hoc* basis, is unclear.

Postgraduate and continuing medical education (see Figure 3.2)

At the undergraduate level, the tensions between the requirements of medical training as defined by the profession and the immediate needs of the service as defined by purchasing agencies are centred on the relationship between universities and Trusts, with the GMC acting as a ringside commentator. At the postgraduate and continuing medical education (CME) level, the situation is more complex, the agencies more numerous and the lines of self-regulation more convoluted (Dowie, 1987). As the pressures for change develop, so they are producing shifts in the balance of power between the regulating agencies in this field.

Historically, the Royal Colleges and Faculties have dominated postgraduate training and CME through their accredition and validation powers. Following their initial training and registration by the GMC as a medical practitioner, doctors undertake basic specialist training (also known as general professional training) for a period of two or three years, acquire a qualification such as Fellow of the Royal College of Surgeons (FRCS – an exit qualification from basic specialist training) or Member of the Royal College of Physicians (MRCP – an entry qualification for higher specialist training) which then allows them to proceed to a further period of higher specialist training of three to five years. Completion of this training is usually attested by accreditation by the Royal Colleges as a specialist or by an 'exit' qualification. Alternatively, following registration they may opt to undertake a three-year period of vocational training for general practice in order to obtain the Certificate of Prescribed/Equivalent Experience issued by the Joint Committee on Postgraduate Training for General Practice under the National Health Service (Vocational Training) regulations 1979 (GMC, Education Committee, 1987: 3; Joint Committee on Higher Medical Training [JCHMT] 1992: 15–16).

Up to 1996 and the implementation of the recommendations of the Calman Report *Hospital Doctors: Training for the Future* following pressure from the European Union, none of these post-graduate training qualifications were linked to a GMC register of fitness to practice (Working Group on Specialist Medical Training, 1993). Nor did a specialist qualification entitle a hospital doctor to consultant status, or its absence necessarily exclude him/her from such status, since the title of consultant was, and is, bestowed by the employer. With the passing by Parliament of the European Specialist Medical Qualifications Order in early 1996, a new regulatory framework was introduced consisting of the UK Certificate of Completion of Specialist Training (CCST), the Specialist Training Authority (STA) and the Specialist Register. The CCST indicates that 'the doctor has satisfactorily completed specialist training, based on assessment of competence, to a standard compatible with independent practice and eligibility for consideration for appointment to a consultant post (*ibid.*: 5). Accreditation of the CCST is awarded by the STA (a joint Colleges–GMC body) on the recommendation of the appropriate Medical Royal College and enables the doctor's name to be included on the Specialist Register which is maintained and published by the GMC. Entry on the Specialist Register (*not* the award of a CCST) makes the doctor eligible to be appointed to an NHS consultant post, subject to the statutory appointment committee procedures, and it is a mandatory requirement to be on the Specialist Register before a doctor can take up a substantive consultant post. A new structure of elite medical power has thus been created, nicely linking the accreditation functions of the Colleges with the standards maintenance funtions of the GMC.

General practitioners as yet remain outside this system. They have to have acquired the Certificate of Prescribed/Equivalent Experience before they can become a principal in a GP practice but do not have to have passed the Royal College of General Practitioners' (RCGP) membership exam (MRCGP). (About 70 per cent of trainees get the MRCGP within twelve months of completing training [Huntington, 1994: 23]).

To be valid, postgraduate training has to take place within an 'approved' junior doctor post: senior house officer (SHO – for general professional and basic specialist training) and specialist registrar (for higher specialist training). 'Each approved post carries an accreditable value – the period of accreditable higher medical training that can be gained in each speciality for which the post is approved' (JCHMT, 1992: 19). For SHOs, the power to validate posts in England, Wales and Northern Ireland rests with the Royal College of Physicians in London, and in Scotland with the Regional Postgraduate Committees. Thereafter, approval of specialist registrar training posts is granted by the JCHMT and its specialist advisory committees acting on behalf of the Royal Colleges. Once approved, posts remain valid for training purposes for up to five years but the JCHMT has to be notified if there is any change of consultant or hospital organisation (for example rotation of junior doctors). In the case of GPs, the accreditation and validation function is carried out by the Joint Committee on Postgraduate Training for General Practice which, unlike the JCHMT, is a statutory body.

Because the large majority of junior doctor posts are 'approved' training posts, Trusts are in the position where they must share control of part of their staffing establishment with the Royal Colleges and, in initiating any change in that workforce, are obliged to operate within procedural constraints determined by those same Colleges. At the same time Trusts have to contend with the growing power of the Postgraduate Deans whose regulating role in several respects duplicates, and to an extent challenges, that of the Royal Colleges to the point where tensions between the two agencies are not unknown (Hann, 1994a).

Jointly appointed by a university and the regional office of the NHSE, the Postgraduate Dean has been an integral part of postgraduate and continuing medical education since the present system was introduced following the Christchurch Conference convened by the Nuffield Provincial Hospitals Trust in 1961. However, of late both the nature of his role and the power behind it have become considerably more robust, and rather less informal, in the wake of the 1989 Review of the NHS. *Working for Patients, Postgraduate and Continuing Medical and Dental Education* made it clear that Deans 'will be charged with the management and control of the financial arrangements for the medical and dental education programmes' and:

> will set the regional educational programme, organise provision of training at regional level where appropriate, monitor the quality of both the education and facilities provided for all grades of staff and encourage the development of rotational training schemes. (NHSME, 1991f: 13)

Furthermore, Deans were to be given a specific budget to add financial power to their elbow. Initially, this was not to include any element of salary costs (which was to remain the responsibility of the Health Authorities (*ibid.*: 5) but with the 1992 circular *The funding of hospital medical and dental training grade posts* a dramatic shift occurred.

The circular asked Regions to establish a budget to cover: 50 per cent of the basic salary costs for all approved posts in the medical and dental training grades (including GP vocational trainees), pre-registration house officers (medical), and post-registration house officers (dental); the full costs of part-time posts in training grades; full-time honorary contract holders where these are fully funded by the NHS; and non-pay costs and travel (NHSE, 1992b, Annex B). As Regions had no idea what postgraduate medical training cost (because like undergraduate medical training it had always been a professionally controlled and non-accountable area of expenditure) this was a tall order. Regional and DHA accounting procedures were not designed to identify separately expenditure on postgraduate medical education (Standing Committee on Postgraduate and Continuing Medical Education [SCOPME], 1990: 27). Unabashed, Regions produced the budgets and by 1993 the Postgraduate Deans were in business.

Under the new regime, Postgraduate Deans are the purchasers and Trusts the providers of medical training. Trusts deliver their medical training service according to the requirements of an annual contract with the Dean. This contract may specify the facilities to be provided, the standards to be achieved, the mandatory achievement of the junior doctors' hours ('New Deal') agreement, and the non-variation of the establishment without the agreement of the Dean (see for example, Medway NHS Trust, 1994). At the local level, the contract is managed and the budget controlled by the Clinical Tutor, a consultant who is both an employee of the Trust and, through a separate contract, accountable to the Dean.

While Royal Colleges can apply pressure to Trusts using their power of validation of posts, Postgraduate Deans are now able to use direct and indirect financial sanctions. This gives them a number of political advantages over the Colleges: the financial lever is more flexible and more effective than the sledgehammer of College withdrawal of recognition and, through the role of the Clinical Tutor, Deans have a management and monitoring presence at the Trust level. Unresolved is the issue of how colleges and Deans are to relate in the future in order to regulate their common territory of medical education. At present they co-exist, with varying degrees of uneasiness, in alliances which work through the regional post-graduate medical education committees, of which the Deans are the chairs. While this informal arrangement has worked in the past, the increasing demands being placed upon the Postgraduate Dean make it inevitable that he will seek to be the dominant partner in the relationship.

The power of the Dean is intended to create a protected enclave for postgraduate medical education within which the provision of high quality training is assured. In his lecture to the Harveian Society in December 1993 Brian Mawhinney, then Minister for Health, quoted the White Paper *Working for Patients*'s statement that Trusts would be given a range of powers and freedoms not available to Health Authorities and commented: 'The overall intention was that NHS Trusts should be free to employ whatever and however many staff they consider necessary. We need to move towards enabling Trusts to exercise the freedom they were promised' (Mawhinney, 1994). How these freedoms to respond to the internal market were to be reconciled with the increasingly specific and contract based requirements of the training enclave was not explained.

For the future, the developments most likely to impact on the relative powers of the regulating agencies in postgraduate and continuing medical education are the full implementation of the Calman Report, with its dramatic reduction of specialist training from twelve to seven years, and the developing issue of continuing medical education. While the introduction of the CCST can be regarded as a long-awaited rationalisation of postgraduate training prompted by pressure from the European Union, the changes to CME are undoubtedly a response to the public's declining confidence in the authority of the medical profession. As the Chief Medical Officer's consultation paper on the subject observes:

> The case for CME rests heavily on the concept of confidence: clinicians must command the confidence of the patients they treat; of the public as a whole; of the hospital managers to whom they are accountable for the quality of service to patients; and NHS managers who contract with hospitals on behalf of patients must have confidence in the quality of service they buy. (Calman, 1994b: 6)

Whereas in previous years the legitimacy of a doctor's clinical competence was assured by the very fact of their having qualified as a medical practitioner, now it is argued that 'a more formal' and continuous system is required to assuage public doubts (*ibid.*). In the first instance it has been the Royal Colleges who have taken the lead in developing a system for controlling this new area of self-regulation. Each is defining the content, the monitoring and certification procedures of CME and the contribution expected from college tutors, clinical tutors, Postgraduate Deans and unit managers.

Two issues remain to be decided before the long-term impact of CME on the balance of power within the medical profession is resolved: the sanctions for non-compliance with CME regulations and the identity of the agency which applies the sanctions. If the sanctions are weak the political significance of CME diminishes accordingly. At present the proposed sanctions of the Colleges vary but none includes the principle of deregistration. The sanctions include: exclusion from being considered for merit awards and college committee membership (Royal College of Gynaecologists), loss of teacher status (Royal College of Opthalmologists), and viewing a consultant without CME accreditation as a reason for the non-approval of training posts with which he is associated (Royal College of Physicians) (Ward, 1994: 18). Such measures are unlikely to achieve the desired effect of improving public confidence in the medical profession and are likely to be replaced by more rigorous measures. Second, which body should hold the register of CME-accredited doctors? While the Colleges may presently see this as their province there have already been suggestions that the function would more naturally sit alongside the other registration functions of the GMC (see for example Calman, 1994b: 11).

The self-regulating mechanisms of medical training and accreditation are beginning to respond to the pressures for change. That they are doing so at all is significant given the traditional inertia in this field in the face of repeated recommendations for reform. Despite the proposals of the Royal Commission on Medical Education in 1968 (the Todd Report), the vigorous restatement of the reform proposals in the Merrison Report on the NHS in 1979 and the report on medical education from the House of Commons Social Services Committee in 1981 (the Short Report), the observable impact on the practices of the medical profession was negligible (Biggs, 1994: 6). As the regulating agencies of medical education progressively recognise that change is required, it is inevitable that some will be better equipped, or positioned, than others to deliver the appropriate response. It follows that a mutual re-evaluation of the historic power relationships between the universities, GMC, Postgraduate Deans and Royal Colleges must take place as part of the hard political bargaining over who should control what. If successful, out of this will emerge a reformulation of the contribution of medical elites to the concordat.

Career structure

The concordat between medicine and the state allowed the profession to determine key aspects of its own career structure. It could influence decisions about the size and make-up of the medical workforce, assume a privileged set of pay and conditions for its senior members, and control its senior appointments and promotions. This arrangement was facilitated by central, state-sponsored planning procedures which the profession dominated and by the absence of any real incentives for NHS managers to oppose it. Into this comfortable situation was injected the destabilizing effects of the 1991 reforms accompanied by growing consumer pressure on doctors for greater accountability and less protection. The logic of these developments is that medicine's control of its own career structure in hospitals will be challenged by Trusts as they seek to manage their medical staff in a way which enables them to meet the demands from purchasing agencies and patients. GPs, meanwhile, will remain their own managers but their career opportunities are likely to depend at least partly on their ability to handle the pressures from that new NHS animal: the merged District Health Authority (DHA) and Family Health Service Authority (FHSA).

Echoing its predecessors, the last major report on medicine's career structure *Achieving a Balance* observed that the underlying problem of hospital medical staffing is the basic conflict between two principles:

> i. that all junior doctors seeking a hospital career are in training for consultant posts and that this training should last no longer than is strictly necessary;
>
> and
>
> ii. that all consultants should have adequate support, for example to cover out-of-hours emergencies and to perform more routine procedures. (DHSS, 1987b: 5)

As the second principle is also a statement about service needs, albeit from the medical profession's viewpoint, it is of interest to learn that 'the requirement for support staff has predominated' and that the number of training posts far exceeds the numbers required to train future consultants (*ibid.*).

The assumption in this and earlier reports, is that a doctor achieves full professional recognition only when he becomes a consultant and that other classes of medical employment are either stations on the road to that destination or, as in the case of GPs, part of a separate, and lower, professional order. All else is seen to flow from this assumption and, in terms of manpower planning, it has always been the dominating theme. From medicine's perspective, therefore, the hospital career hierarchy is essentially a training hierarchy and should be organised accordingly. Hence we find reports on the medical workforce in the NHS focus on the relationship between junior doctor and consultant numbers and recommend either restricting the former, or expanding the latter, or both in order to produce a balanced supply of future consultants (*ibid.*: 6). Only the Short Report of 1981 on medical education took the unusual view that the fundamental issue should be the quality of patient care, not the careers of doctors (*ibid.*: 7). In general the unchallenged principle was 'that doctors should not be unduly delayed in their progression through the training system' (*ibid.*: 87).

Despite the assiduously propagated view of the NHS as a vehicle for medical training to consultant level, the reality has always been one where, ultimately, service needs could neither be wholly ignored nor forced into the pint bottle of training requirements. There have always been more SHO posts than are needed for training purposes (Isaacs, 1993) and SHOs and registrars have frequently become 'stuck', as it is known, at some point along the long road to consultant status, effectively providing what the Royal College of Surgeons has called 'a sub-consultant service' (Royal College of Surgeons of England, 1988: 5). Associate specialist and staff grade appointments have acted as tactfully disguised support for this sub-consultant service in order to sustain the profession's political ambitions as well as its pride. But with the 1991 reforms giving an extra contract-based edge to service-led demand and the Calman proposals producing qualified specialists without the experience traditionally expected of consultants, it is doubtful whether the illusion can be sustained much longer.

Further distortions in the training–service equation are bound to result from the progressive reduction in junior doctors' hours introduced as part of the New Deal agreement (NHSME, 1991g). For the agreement to be implemented fresh junior doctor posts have had to be created which, as well as imposing an extra cost on hospital providers, have stretched the tolerance of the existing pattern of training arrangements to the limit (Hann, 1994b). Once it is publicly recognised that the limit has been exceeded the choice is then between the Royal Colleges declaring the non-training SHO posts to be illegal or redefining them as part of a sub-consultant service. Given that these pressures have now made a rationalisation of the present position an urgent imperative, from medicine's perspective the issue is what levers it can use to influence the reformulation of the training–service relationship which must take place.

Part of the concordat is that the medical profession should shape the parameters of its own career structure by determining the numbers and types of doctors which journey through it. Beginning in 1984 the central planning function was carried out by the Joint Planning Advisory Committee (JPAC) which had 24 members, 20 of whom were doctors (DHSS, 1987b: 86). Until the abolition of the Regional Health Authorities (RHAs) in 1995, the results of JPAC's deliberations were channelled through the Regional Manpower Committees (RMCs), each of which had 11 members and all of whom were doctors (*ibid.*: 89). Despite the structural neatness of this medical hegemony, there is reason to suppose that it was always less than an effective instrument for protecting medicine's view of the professional career structure. In his speech on medical staffing policies to the Harveian Society in 1994, Brian Mawhinney, then Minister for Health, listed a number of problems with the central planning of medical manpower which seriously challenged its effectiveness. He noted that: there were major distributional anomalies in PRHO posts; SHO ceilings were never a reality and were arbitrarily set in the first place; the number of registrar posts has increased despite the recommendations of *Achieving a Balance* that they should reduce; the failure to plan senior registrar posts effectively means that there are renewed shortages of candidates for new consultant posts in some key specialties; and the central funding for consultants has not always provided an appropriate specialist balance (Mawhinney, 1994). By 1995 there was a general recognition that not enough doctors were being trained and the decision was taken to increase the target intake of medical schools by 10 per cent from 4 470 to 4 970 by the year 2000 (Warden, 1995b; see also Medical Workforce Standing Advisory Committee, 1995).

Given what one suspects is an historic failure of medical manpower planning, presided over and disguised by committees dominated by the profession itself, there is little reason to suppose that these same committees will be able to resist the redistributive pressures now generated by the internal market. The recent demise of JPAC and its replacement by the Advisory Group on Medical Education, Training and Staffing (AGMETS), which has purely a monitoring role, is a recognition that, as the Medical Manpower Standing Advisory Committee (MMSAC) observed, 'increasingly, purchasers will control the manpower agenda by deciding which services are bought' (MMSAC, 1992: 14). There remains, of course, the Postgraduate Dean as a barrier to such service pressures and as a champion of medicine's traditional career rights. Given that this is a joint appointment by Region and University, the Dean is likely to experience acute role conflict as he seeks to resolve the tensions between, on the one hand, his management accountability to the Region and NHS Executive and, on the other, his responsibility to his professional colleagues. Already the signs are that he will be sorely tested. The medical manpower figures for 1992–3 show that compared to the previous year the number of consultants grew by 1.9 per cent, senior registrars by 4.2 per cent, SHOs by 5 per cent and, significantly, staff grade appointments by 50 per cent (Brearley, 1994: 1245). Such a dramatic increase in non-career grade, sub-consultant appointments is clearly a challenge to medicine's traditional view of its career structure.

While the ability of the profession to resist demands for a reshaping of its overall grade structure must be regarded as suspect, this could be at least partly offset by a comprehensive control of individual appointments and promotions. Up to the level of specialist registrar a doctor's career progress is largely governed by the Royal Colleges (as the accrediting agencies) and by appointments procedures with a joint clinician–management composition. Thereafter, the appointment of registrars and consultants is a matter guided by statutory instruments which stipulate the composition of the Advisory Appointment Committees (AACs). These instruments make clear that although the make-up of the committees may vary according to certain rules, professional members are always to be in the majority (DoH, 1989b; NHSME, 1991h). On the medical side there will generally be representation from the Royal Colleges, University and Postgraduate Dean and, on the Trust side, from the Trust Board. In technical terms the management presence, though not dominant, is substantial enough to restrict the operation of medical power. But whether management is sophisticated enough to deal with the long-established and informal networks of medical influence over appointments is less certain (see Allen, 1988, 1994).

In general practice, the career progress of a doctor remains very much in the hands of his/her colleagues. Since 1948, applications from doctors to set up in practice have been authorized by the national Medical Practices Committee (made up entirely of doctors) using a strict doctor:population ratio to determine whether or not a town or district is 'open', 'restricted' or 'closed' (Moran and Wood, 1993: 49). Appointments to existing practices are solely a matter for the GP or partners concerned.

Within the NHS, the remuneration of doctors is subject to national pay scales which, while not a part of the profession's self-regulating functions, can nonetheless be regarded as embedded within its sphere of influence as part of the concordat arrangements. The long-established procedure is that the BMA negotiates with the Secretary of State about the structure of the payment system and the Review Body on Doctors and Dentists Remuneration (known as the DDRB) gives a monetary interpretation to this system which the government duly accepts. It was a logical part of a market approach to the NHS that this state-sponsored arrangement should give way to a system of local pay bargaining capable of responding to the ebb and flow of demand for medical manpower and all Trusts were obliged to have local pay machinery set up by February 1995. Clearly such a system might have made it more difficult for the profession to retain control of part of its own reward structure. On the other hand, the medical profession's remunerative relationship with the private sector is already fairly fluid. Although GPs operate within a recommended schedule of fees set by the BMA, hospital consultants do not and the only regulatory activity in their case is carried out by the insurance companies – with no apparent complaints from doctors. In short it may well be that the profession had nothing to fear from local pay bargaining and that market dominance through the monopoly of scarce skills is, and will be, a more than adequate substitute for state-sponsored pay scales. In any case, few Trusts chose to change their consultants' contracts and those that did made only minimal changes (Moore, 1995: 24).

Beyond the consultant level, further progress in medicine's career structure is through the merit award system introduced as part of the

1948 concordat package and traditionally an undisputed realm of medical influence. Up to 1996, the system had four levels ranging from a 'C' award to an 'A+' award (which can double a clinician's salary) and in applying for an award clinicians were judged on their research, clinical excellence, teaching and, for 'C' awards, management effort (Chadda, 1994). Given the not insubstantial sums involved, the emerging problem for Trusts in a situation where consultant costs necessarily form part of the pricing equation is whether Trust managements have any influence over the merit award decisions which impact on the cost base of their organisations (Hern, 1994: 173). To an extent, from 1996 the problem was alleviated by the government decision that there should be two types of merit award. 'A' and 'B' awards were to continue to be nationally determined and centrally funded and 'C' awards were replaced by a discretionary awards scheme with the costs borne by the Trust employers. Although management representation on the central Advisory Committee on Distinction Awards (ACDA) and the regional subcommittees for national awards has been increased to a quarter of the membership, medicine retains its dominance. Meanwhile the profession constitutes 60 per cent of the local awards committees. These receive nominations from employers following consultation with their consultants (Beecham, 1994: 1187). However, whether these new arrangments will allow management to link merit awards to clinical performance, and so affect a revolution in consultant accountability to their employers, remains to be seen. What is certain is that medicine's control of this particular territory will not be lightly conceded.

All in all it is a useful, though probably short-term, political fudge which leaves medicine's professional hold on promotions through the system of peer review more or less intact. Whether it will survive in this form depends to an extent on how far Trusts are able to take advantage of their notional rights to negotiate new pay arrangements and employment conditions with their consultants now that they hold the consultant contracts previously held by Region (see for example, Clark and Gray, 1994). If this option is seriously exploited and the position of the national Review Body on Doctors' and Dentists' Remuneration undermined, local incentive systems controlled by management could eventually replace the merit award system. Given the secure market position of senior doctors, however, this may simply mean that consultants get paid more.

Professional standards

It was no coincidence that the 1858 Medical Act, the initial bargain between medicine and the state, gave the medical profession the right and the duty to determine and regulate its own professional standards. For in this principle lies the very core of a profession's identity and the source of its internal loyalty and cohesion. The mechanism chosen was the General Medical Council (GMC), financed by the profession itself and answerable to Parliament through the Privy Council. Subsequently, as part of the 1948 concordat and the foundation of the NHS, other purely NHS procedures have been introduced which in some respects parallel, and in others, duplicate those of the GMC. In effect, two mechanisms for regulating professional standards have been created: one directly controlled by the profession and one indirectly through the medium of the NHS. For the profession to retain the respect of an increasingly sceptical public while responding to the internal market's demands for clinical performance of an demonstrably acceptable standard, it will need to show that these existing procedures, or an amended version of them, constitute a legitimate means of self-regulation.

The GMC controls entry to, and exit from, the profession by maintaining a register of doctors fit to practise medicine. Following successful completion of the pre-registration year, an individual's name is entered on the Register and can be removed only if the GMC's Professional Conduct Committee judges him guilty of 'serious professional misconduct' (GMC, 1993). Although the Council also deals with sick doctors through the work of its Health Committee, this Committee does not have the power of erasure if it deems a doctor's fitness to practise to be seriously impaired. It can, however, suspend, or impose conditions upon, a doctor's registration (*ibid.*: 42). Finally, the Council has the power to provide advice for members of the profession on standards of professional conduct or medical ethics and it has the educational functions discussed earlier.

As one would expect of a body which is central to the self-regulating ethos of the medicine–state concordat, the membership of the Council is almost exclusively medical (Stacey, 1984: 25). In the present context, from the state's perspective the question is whether an organisational solution to a nineteenth-century problem is still appropriate in the context of a different health care system, in a changed society generating different political demands. For the most part, the reforms of the GMC have thus far served to reconcile the various medical factions rather than to reassure the public that the profession can guarantee the maintenance of satisfactory standards among its membership (Smith, 1989a: 1300) – the original purpose of the GMC. Its procedures are lengthy and cumbersome while its sanctions are draconian and, in consequence, seldom used. Hence as a result of a total of 1615 complaints received in 1992–93, 13 doctors were suspended and 30 erased from the register (GMC, 1994: 14–18).

If the political utility and legitimacy of the GMC as a self-regulating instrument is to be retained, it must address the issue of how it reverses the decline of public confidence in the profession. Complaints to the GMC are increasing at an impressive rate. In the year 1991–92 they rose by 20 per cent and in 1992–93 by a further 24 per cent (*ibid.*: 14). In this context, if the Council's new procedures for dealing with the long-term poor performance of doctors are to be successful, these procedures will have to convince the public that the profession can insist on the maintenance of particular standards among its members (Smith, 1992). The GMC is clearly aware of the problem. In 1995 its new President Sir Donald Irvine identified its key problem as 'getting its image and its relationship right with the outside world'. He continued, 'It must be seen to be interested in good practice and to be connecting with patients' concerns. It shouldn't be seen simply as a punitive body that does or doesn't work depending on your point of view' (Smith, 1995b: 1515). As part of this new approach the Council has issued the booklet *Good Medical Practice* as guidance on the principles of good professional practice. However, there is a cost to this move from its traditional reactive style – where it responds to complaints from the police, NHS, public and doctors – to a more pro-active stance and a limit to how much can be achieved. Even the responsive style placed considerable strain on its resources. The GMC is financed through its registration fee and while reform may be desirable it has to be recognised, as Smith observes, that 'doctors will pay so much for the privilege of self-regulation but would probably be unwilling to pay the several hundred pounds a year that might be required for a more intensive and extensive disciplinary system' (Smith, 1989b: 1504). The balance between the need to reassure the public that standards are being maintained, on the one hand, and the cost to the profession of such measures, on the other, is a delicate one to strike and will almost certainly require a measure of support from the state.

As the profession moves to redefine this part of the concordat, its difficulties are compounded by the fact that other aspects of professional standards are dealt with by the NHS's three categories of disciplinary procedures: personal misconduct, professional misconduct and professional incompetence. Personal misconduct, such as assault or sexual harassment, falls within the remit of the employer's internal disciplinary procedures. Professional misconduct or incompetence involving the exercise of clinical skills, however, are accorded a separate disciplinary status to that of other NHS employees and are dealt with by a complex set of procedures contained in two government circulars (DHSS, 1982; DoH, 1990b). The procedures invoked under the guidance of these circulars are either, in the less serious cases, a form of peer review or, where they could result in dismissal, are in the words of the only formal study of this issue: 'legalistic, time consuming, expensive, and intimidating to those who might wish to report a problem or who might have something relevant to say on the matter' (Donaldson, 1994a: 1281). Further problems in implementing the procedures arise from the difficulty of establishing a clinician's precise contractual responsibilities against which to measure performance, the automatic closing of ranks by a doctor's peer group and, in the case of sick doctors, reluctance on the part of doctors to activate a procedure with disciplinary connotations (*ibid.*: 1280; Donaldson, 1994b).

The use of disciplinary procedures to maintain professional standards assumes that the disciplining body is dealing with exceptions to a general rule of good practice. An alternative view now beginning to assert itself within medicine is that this good practice cannot be assumed but should be actively promoted by the profession, albeit within the constraints of clinical autonomy. From this perspective the developments in medical audit (see for example, Royal College of Physicians of London, 1989; Royal College of Surgeons of England, 1989), continuing medical education, evidence-based medicine (see for example, Delamothe, 1994), and information bases such as the National Confidential Enquiry into Perioperative Deaths (see for example, Campling *et al.*, 1992) are part of a growing awareness that explicit self-monitoring with formal backing from professional bodies such as the Royal Colleges is both necessary and politically desirable. So far the state has taken the view that the terms of the concordat should be respected and that the profession should remain responsible for the quality of the service it delivers. Thus *Working for Patients*, while insisting that every district should have a medical audit committee, also reaffirmed that 'the quality of medical work should be reviewed by a doctor's peers' (DoH, 1989a: 40). Ringfenced money was subsequently made available to support and encourage the profession's acceptance of self-audit. Given the overlap between this arrangement and the existing tenor of the concordat it is not surprising to learn that medical audit was just about the only part of the reforms package on which the DoH and the national bodies of medicine were in broad agreement (Harrison *et al.*, 1992: 142).

What remains unresolved, however, is what the profession should do about those of its members who are shown to be poor performers or who resist monitoring altogether. What, for example, should be the relationship between local audit and any performance monitoring procedures introduced by the GMC (Smith, 1992: 1258)? If self-monitoring is able to detect poor professional standards but if the self-correcting mechanisms are weak, variable or absent, public confidence in the profession may actually decline as a result of this new openness.

Conclusions

The 1948 concordat between medicine and the state was a high level political agreement with advantages to both parties. For the state it provided a means for controlling the ever-increasing demand for health care engendered by the principles of the welfare state. For medicine it meant an enhanced ability to regulate its own professional affairs coupled with economic security and a key role in the disposal of NHS resources: its existing professional autonomy was thus complemented by political and economic autonomy. Unchanged for 50 years, the concordat is in need of serious revision if its considerable political utility to both sides is to be retained.

A number of pressures have combined to render reform essential. Medicine's negotiating power has always been founded on the twin assumptions that it has unique access to medical knowledge and that it is regarded by the public as the legitimate purveyor of medical wisdom. In today's society both of these assumptions are questionable and, in consequence, the basis of medical power is no longer as secure as it once was. If public confidence in medical decision-making is less absolute, it follows that the ability of the profession to define and ration the demand for health care is reduced and, correspondingly, so is its political usefulness to the state. With its bargaining power thus diminished, medicine should be more amenable to suggestions for a renegotiation of the concordat – always assuming, of course, that it notices its theoretical loss of power.

Within the NHS, the logic of the 1991 reforms has been to challenge the clinical and political autonomy of doctors while, as yet, leaving the economic autonomy of their remuneration and reward systems undisturbed. Hospital medical staff are under increasing pressure from their employing Trust to tailor their clinical and resource-allocating decisions to the corporate needs of the Trust as these are reflected in the flow of contracts from purchasing agencies. Not to do so puts the income and, ultimately, the survival of the organisation at risk. At present, the historic right of the medical profession to regulate its own training and accreditation, career progress and maintenance of professional standards means that Trusts lack the means to insist that the corporate interest is put above that of the profession where the two conflict. Clearly the logic of the reforms is that Trusts should try and develop such means, presumably with support from the state, and herein lie the specifics of the challenge to the concordat.

If the medical profession chooses to respond to this challenge by employing its normal, negative power tactic of blocking change until the political pressure has evaporated it will merely postpone the evil day of reckoning. Inaction may stymie the 1991 reforms but it will not deal with the problem of public confidence in the profession.

The alternative strategy is that the profession actively seeks to redefine its own mechanisms of self-regulation in order both to re-establish its legitimacy in the eyes of the public and to reach an accommodation with the reforms. There are two major problems with this option which, while not insuperable, require the profession to develop quite novel forms of political skills and organisation if the obstacles are to be overcome. First, this chapter has shown the fragmented, not to say haphazard, system of self-regulation evolved by a profession which has never had to suffer the ignominy of an externally imposed settlement. Left to its own devices by a state held hostage by its own promises to the citizenry, medicine has simply perpetuated the historic divisions between its constituent power centres of Royal Colleges, GMC and Universities and occasionally added another layer of medical power within the NHS bureaucracy (for example, Postgraduate Deans). The result has been duplication of function, confused lines of accountability, inter-institutional rivalries and, not surprisingly, dilution of effect.

Given the absence of any coordinating body with the authority to resolve these inefficiencies, a way forward has to be invented acceptable to the major power groups concerned. Essentially, then, the second problem is one of elite negotiation within the profession as a mechanism for managing change. The negotiations are bound to be lengthy because not only does a set of agreements have to be reached about the future regulation of medical education, the career structure and professional standards but, within each of these, the redistribution of elite power. There can be little doubt that once elite accommodation on a particular issue is reached it will require rather more formal and public sanction than has been the practice in the past. To quote some examples, in order that the CCST could be accredited by the Royal Colleges, awarded by the STA and linked to a Specialist Register of fitness to practice held and maintained by the GMC, parliamentary sanction was essential. And, if the Postgraduate Dean's role of monitoring postgraduate training on behalf of the Region is to be properly squared with Royal College responsibilities, the division of labour between the two will have to be carefully identified. Finally, if the GMC is to play a part in promoting improved medical performance it will have to find a way of relating to the range of quality monitoring activities already established.

Assuming that a new style of elite alliances is adopted by medicine as a way of redefining and maintaining the concordat with the state, this must have an impact on the internal dynamics of the profession. The price of improved regulation mechanisms will be an expansion of elite power and a diminution of individual doctors' freedoms. While the medical profession as a whole will retain its clinical, political and economic autonomy (albeit in amended form), the price will be a tightened and more effective control over its internal affairs and the activities of its individual members. It is only through putting its own house in order that medicine will enable the concordat between itself and the state to survive and prosper.

The state, meanwhile, is in an ambiguous position. It has initiated reforms which place pressure on the concordat yet it is not in the state's interest for the concordat to be dismantled. If this were to happen, the state would find itself directly confronted with the results of the plethora of social rights it has given its citizens: an infinite demand for health care. Since the state relies on the medical profession to control that demand it must, ultimately, support the profession in its attempts to redefine the concordat. It can prod, nudge and offer encouragement but otherwise its hands are tied. It may have divided the profession and rocked its status hierarchy by giving GP Fundholders exceptional powers, but the state cannot rule.

6

Nursing

Introduction

Unlike medicine, nursing exercises little control over the demand for health care. Its political utility to a state striving to deal with the ever-rising curve of citizen expectations is therefore minimal and, in this respect, its bargaining position in the grand politics of welfare is inherently weak. Nursing will never rival medicine and have its own concordat with the state (see Chapter 5). Nevertheless, against this it can be argued that within the NHS nursing is not without power because it is the largest single occupation, it has some measure of professional autonomy, it is historically deeply embedded in Health Service structures and in times of crisis it is able to call upon substantial public sympathy.

In exploring nursing's contribution to the politics of change in the NHS, this chapter begins by analysing the basis of its historic relationship with the medical profession and the inherent constraints which lie therein. Second, it examines the attempts by the nursing profession to challenge this relationship, to improve both its status and its power base in the Health Service and the consequences, intended and unintended, of this manoeuvering. Third, it deals with the impact of successive government policies on nursing's ambitions and the realignment of power relations which has followed.

Nursing and medicine

Nursing exists within a state-sponsored system of medical hegemony. As a result of the 1948 concordat between medicine and the state, the medical profession was given clinical, economic and political autonomy within the NHS on condition that it arranged a continuing accommodation between patient demand and the health care resources available. While this bargain continues to deliver its benefits to both parties, nursing must necessarily enjoy a subordinate political status to the logic of the bargain and, therefore, to the position of medicine.

Traditionally, this subordinate status was apparent in the contribution made by nursing to the key areas of medical decision-making which determine a patient's progress through a course of NHS treatment: diagnosis, admission, treatment plan, treatment delivery, and discharge. Through these decisions a doctor determines how many patients are treated, for how long, and at what cost: in other words, the demands placed upon the Health Service. This professional dominance was, and is, reinforced by the legal position. The consultant, or the principal in general practice, is legally responsible and accountable for the care and well-being of his/her patients and for ensuring that the delegation of tasks to others such as nursing is appropriate (see for example, Montgomery, 1992). Failure properly to fulfil this responsibility exposes the doctor to charges of negligence. Hence, as a professional safeguard, the General Medical Council (GMC) guidelines on the delegation of tasks to nurses emphasise the ultimate responsibility of the doctor, the need to be satisfied about the competence of nurses, and the fact that improper delegation renders the doctor liable to disciplinary procedings (Witz, 1994: 34).

In this context, the traditional role of the nurse is that of 'handmaiden' to the doctor. The doctor determines the treatment to be carried out and the nurse delivers it under medical supervision. Any change in the treatment requires medical authorisation in order to protect the doctor in any subsequent negligence inquiry. Regardless of nursing's ambitions, of which more later, this remains the formal position and any delegation to, or discretion exercised by, the nurse should technically occur within the orbit of medical control. Until comparatively recently, the customary approach of the nursing profession was to accept the constraints imposed by the medical hegemony, to work within them and to develop the nursing role under the umbrella of medical protection. Thus *The Duties and Position of the Nurse*, a joint publication by the Royal College of Nursing (RCN) and the British Medical Association (BMA) (first published in 1961 and revised several times thereafter up to 1978), recognised that the scope of nursing practice would have to change as the result of advances in medical science and the introduction of new techniques. It proposed that in order to safeguard the professional position of the nurse joint committees of medical and nursing staff should be set up on a local basis to oversee 'the increasing responsibility devolved on the nurse carrying out these new forms of treatment' (*ibid.*).

In due course, this inter-professional agreement received state support through the Department of Health and Social Security (DHSS) circular *The extending role of the nurse – legal implications and training requirements* (DHSS, 1977). The circular approvingly quoted the Briggs Report's observation regarding 'the essential differences between the caring role of nurses and the diagnostic and curative function of doctors' but made clear that 'where delegation occurs, the doctor remains responsible for his patient and for the overall management of treatment, and the nurse is responsible for carrying out delegated tasks competently' (*ibid.*: 2). To ensure that this happened, work ought to be delegated to nurses only where:

> (a) the nurse has been specifically and adequately trained for the new task, (b) the training has been recognised as satisfactory by the employing Authority, (c) the new task has been recognised by the profession and by the employing Authority as a task which may be properly delegated to a nurse, (d) *the delegating doctor has been assured of the competence of the individual nurse concerned.* (*ibid.*: emphasis added)

By this means the state confirmed and legitimised a medically dominated hierarchy of delegation and control in the NHS workplace. Further, it ensured that any changes in the boundary between the two professions could occur only with the consent of the doctors.

As one would expect, behind this arrangement lay certain assumptions concerning the respective autonomies and competences of nursing and medicine. Two occupational groups so closely involved in the delivery of patient care could not, it was assumed, enjoy equal amounts of autonomy. Medicine's clinical and political autonomy, supported by the state, to dispose of NHS resources as it saw fit meant that nursing must subordinate its own professional identity to that autonomy. So although nursing was allowed to enjoy some autonomy and discretion in the workplace, this was assumed to be only with the agreement of the medical profession. Equally, while the clinical autonomy of doctors assumed the individual to have a general professional competence and to require no further formal training, any change in the role of the nurse through the acquisition of additional competences was deemed to require accreditation.

The preparedness of the nursing profession to accommodate itself to the conditions of medical autonomy had its advantages. Nursing effectively became a protectorate within the medical sphere of influence and for several decades benefited from the stability and inertia of the institutional arrangements in which it was ensconced. Its numbers steadily increased, its budgets were ringfenced, and it was afforded a measure of self-regulation in the fields of training and professional conduct which, while not directly comparable with the autonomy of medicine, nonetheless represented a qualified recognition by the state of nursing's professional status.

As tangible evidence of this, in 1979 the Nurses, Midwives and Health Visitors Act replaced the General Nursing Council (GNC) with the United Kingdom Central Council for Nursing, Midwifery and Health Visiting (UKCC) and the four National Boards for England, Wales, Scotland and Northern Ireland which, together, gave nursing an enhanced degree of professional self-control. (The governing bodies of both UKCC and National Boards are composed almost exclusively of qualified nurses.) In the field of education and training, the UKCC has the task of determining the policies, embodied as rules in statutory instruments, which will ensure that the minimum standards are met for admission to the register of qualified nurses held by the Council. It specifies the entry requirements for nurse training courses, the length of the course, the areas of practice and the competencies which a person must satisfy if she/he is to be admitted to the register. Working within these policies and requirements, the Boards provide, or arrange for others to provide, courses for training for registration and further training for those already registered. (As we see later, these responsibilities were redefined in 1992.) They hold the powers of validation of courses and the accreditation of institutions and, until 1992, also held the budget for nurse teacher salaries and teacher training. Second, in the field of professional conduct, the Boards investigate instances of alleged misconduct and the Council is responsible for proving misconduct and taking the appropriate action against the nurse, including removal from the register.

From the *Report of the Committee on Senior Nursing Staff* (Salmon Report) in 1968 to the general management reforms of 1985, nursing also enjoyed a degree of self-management which, whilst never independent of the medical hegemony, provided a bulwark against its more ambitious inroads. Salmon gave the profession an exclusive line management structure through the ward sister, nursing officer, senior nurse officer, principal nurse officer to the district nursing officer (Ministry of Health, 1966). At the same time, at district, area (from 1974 to 1982) and regional levels, the chief officers of nursing were given organisational equality with the other NHS management functions such as finance, administration and community medicine and, at district level, generally controlled about a third of the total budget (West, 1992: 53).

Whilst nursing accepted the pre-eminence of medicine in the NHS arena and remained sensitive to the terms of the concordat between medicine and the state, the state for its part was prepared to enhance nursing's professional status within certain limits. Those limits recognised that should the demands of nursing threaten the concordat either in principle or in detail then the profession would find itself dangerously exposed and denuded of state support. Since the foundation of the Health Service, nursing's primary political utility to the state lay in its provision of a large, relatively inexpensive workforce which supported the demand–control activities of the doctors. Its national organisations, such as the Royal College of Nursing (RCN), have never penetrated the elite networks linking medicine and the state nor have they established their own networks but have remained outsiders who derive their strength from their mass membership base (Hart, 1994: Ch. 6). In the absence of any real capacity for, or experience of, elite negotiations over sustained periods of time, mounting a challenge to the medical hegemony was always going to be a risky business. Yet this is what sections of the profession chose to do.

Although the various elements of nursing's challenge emerged at different times with different labels, the overall effect has been to lay claim to a measure of clinical, political and economic autonomy which, if fully implemented, is not compatible with the existing medical dominance of the NHS. As we shall see, medicine has responded to the challenge by offering certain concessions which leave its hegemony intact. In the main, nursing has chosen to ignore these concessions in pursuit of its higher goals.

In order to advance its claim for clinical autonomy, nursing had first to establish its unique contribution to patient health. The main vehicle for this ambitious move has been the concept of 'the nursing process'. Originally developed in the United States in the 1960s, the nursing process sets out a systematic method for identifying patients' problems, developing plans to resolve them, implementing the plans, and evaluating whether they have been effective (Yura and

Walsh, 1978). As this is precisely what doctors claim to do, though they use different terminology, nursing had also to make clear the differences between the two professional approaches. It became necessary to assert that nursing is a therapy in its own right, rather than simply an adjunct to the medical activity, with its own distinctive knowledge base (Henderson, 1966). Hence Baroness Macfarlane, an early champion of the nursing process, maintained that 'the nurse is the authority on the maintenance of daily living activities while the doctor is, for instance [*sic*], the authority on the diagnosis and treatment of disease' (Baroness Macfarlane of Llandaff and Castledine, 1982: 47; see also Aggleton and Chalmers, 1986). She continued, 'The roles are complementary and so closely related as to prohibit an adversarial relationship' (*ibid.*). However, while the distinction between the daily living focus of the nurse and the disease orientation of the doctor may have been unproblematic for the Baroness, for others it raised key issues about who has what power in the nurse–patient–doctor triangle.

For nurses wishing to shrug off the yoke of medical oppression the nursing process established the centrality of clinical nursing in patient care and the means whereby the nurse could claim to have her/his own unique and private relationship with the patient (Witz 1994). The RCN, for one, was clear that 'only professional nurses could set standards and assess and measure the quality of care given' and that 'doctors and nurses must both recognise that their goals for a patient may differ or even conflict' (RCN, 1981). From the beginning, some doctors did recognise this and objected strongly to the invasion of what they saw as their territory. Mitchell argued that because the legal buck stops with the consultant or principal in general practice to whose care the patient has been entrusted, problems will arise if 'there are nursing documents, subserving a nursing diagnosis and a nursing plan, which are independent of or even in opposition to the medical diagnosis and the medical plan'. He concluded 'I do not believe that two people can be equally in charge of one patient' (Mitchell, 1984: 219).

Here was the crux of the matter. Who has control over the patient and, therefore, over the key political area of patient demand? If nursing could install its own relationship with patient demand, independent of the medical hegemony, then it would have the basis for serious elite negotiations with the state. Once it was able to make independent clinical decisions which significantly affected the distribution of NHS resources then it would have achieved a measure of both clinical and political autonomy. Equally, if medicine allowed this to happen then its political monopoly of demand control in the NHS and its concordat with the state would be undermined. Nursing's implementation of the nursing process, and hence of its challenge to medicine, can be examined at the levels of practice and policy.

Practice innovations

The innovations in practice stimulated by the nursing process have generally been local and uncoordinated and have appeared as nurse development units (NDUs), primary nursing and nurse practitioners.

Carried to its logical conclusion, the view of nursing as a therapeutic activity in its own right requires that this therapy should be delivered in a separate unit with nurses given autonomy and accountability for the provision of nursing care. This is because the therapeutic dimension of nursing is deemed to be undermined in acute care settings where the high level of technological and paramedical interventions prevent nurses from focusing on their 'core' nursing roles of caring and nurturing (Pearson *et al.*, 1992). In pursuance of the 'pure' nursing environment, the Oxford and Burford NDUs were established in the mid-1980s where nurses were given the freedom to run their own wards as they saw fit (Pearson 1988, 1992). The continued existence of these NDUs, however, was always dependent upon the sympathy, or indifference, of the local medical profession and once this evaporated the units were duly closed. A more recent example, the Byron Ward Nursing Development Unit at King's Healthcare NHS Trust, has a rather greater chance of longer term success precisely because it has secured the support of its local consultants and its nurses concede that when they receive them their patients are 'medically stable' – that is, the medical episode has finished and the doctors' interest has waned (Griffiths and Evans, 1995).

Although the proponents of what is sometimes described as the 'carative' rather than the 'curative' approach to healing are agreed on the principle of nursing as therapy, disagreements exist around how that therapy is to be delivered. Basically the divide is between (a) those who view the nurse as personally delivering 'holistic' care to meet the full range of potential patient need from toileting and bathing to the more skilled scientific tasks; and (b) those who believe the nurse should concentrate on her/his therapeutic relationship with the patient and, in the time-honoured fashion of the aspirant professional, delegate the more basic tasks to support workers under her supervision (Salvage, 1992). In its more evolved form the latter approach led to the concept of 'primary nursing' where one nurse is responsible and accountable for all the decisions about the nursing care provided on a 24-hour basis for a group of named patients (their primary patients) for the duration of the patients' stay in hospital (Hart, 1994: 150–2). In order to deliver this service the primary nurse manages a team of associate nurses or support workers and this has drawn criticism from other parts of the nursing profession as well as from doctors. For those who believe in personalised holistic nursing, primary nursing's reliance on the management of lower grades of carers suggests an ill-considered elitism which distances the nurse from the patient, which erodes the close nurse–patient relationship on which the nursing therapy depends and which will lead to a profession divided between a core of elite clinical nurses and a mass of associate nurses (see for example, Carpenter, 1977; Robinson, 1992). Over time, it is argued, the associate nurses will be submerged in the new army of National Vocational Qualification (NVQ) qualified support workers leaving the profession consisting of an exposed rump of the clinical nursing elite (Robinson, 1992: 36).

For doctors the concerns are different. The consequences of the primary nursing approach is that the line management structure is flattened out and the traditional hierarchy on which the doctor relies subverted. Instead of dealing with one ward sister the consultant has to weave his/her way through several primary nurses each of whom should, in theory at least, be working to *their* own care plans for the consultant's patients (Hart, 1994: 151; Walby *et al.*, 1994: 34). From the nurse's viewpoint this arrangement protects their ability to design and implement the nursing process but from the doctor's perspective it inhibits the efficient delegation of tasks. It is a situation ripe with potential conflict.

The third form of practice innovation in which the concept of the nursing process has played a significant role is that of the nurse practitioner. Its origins lie in the American experience where a new type of nursing role was developed in response to inadequate medical cover in deprived and rural areas (Bliss and Cohen, 1977). But whereas in the United States nurse practitioners were conceived as a form of doctor substitution in a defined set of non-acute patient conditions, in the UK they have taken on the mantle of the champions of nurse autonomy. Hence we find in Stilwell's description of the nurse practitioner a definition redolent of the nursing process:

> The Nurse Practitioner in primary care settings practises an advanced nursing role and makes professionally autonomous decisions, taking sole responsibility. She/he receives clients with undifferentiated, undiagnosed problems. She/he diagnoses, prescribes and provides care, works closely with other professionals and respects professional boundaries. (Stilwell, 1987: 155)

And in the same vein Pickersgill emphasises that the nurse practitioner 'should be able to make decisions in relation to the assessment and treatment of patients, carry his or her own caseload as well as make and receive referrals from other health professionals' (Pickersgill, 1995: 26). However, while the theory of the nurse practitioner easily embodies the desired status of clinical and political autonomy, the practice is rather different and can perhaps best be described as an autonomy contingent upon medical tolerance.

For the most part, the developments in the nurse practitioner role have occurred sporadically and unofficially (Read *et al.*, 1992: 1469). Accident and Emergency (A and E) Departments are the most common site for the more autonomous nurse practitioner roles where they generally provide an initial assessment function and, in some cases, minor injury treatment (Morris *et al.*, 1989; Potter, 1990; Read and George, 1994). Although it can be rightly argued that the nurse is here dealing with previously unscreened patients and therefore acting in a diagnostic and hence demand-control capacity, the posts are either initiated or sanctioned by the A and E consultants and circumscribed by a negotiated set of protocols.

In other situations the absence of an official definition of the nurse practitioner has led to the proliferation of nursing roles which whilst they may be 'advanced', in the sense that they are beyond what is customarily accepted as the registered nurse role, do not give the nurse the contingent autonomy with unscreened patients which some nurse practitioners enjoy in A and E departments but a delegated task following the doctor's diagnosis. Their titles range from that of nurse practitioner itself to clinical nurse specialist, pre-operative assessment nurse, pre-admission nurse and liaison nurse (see for example Graineer, 1995; Garbett, 1996; Newton, 1996). In general they are, and have always been, responses within medical specialisms to pressures on the workloads of doctors. Traditional examples of this type of role are the diabetes, rheumatology and respiratory nurses. Even if elements of the nursing process survive within these roles, they are clearly subordinate to the medical workload imperatives which have caused the roles to be created in the first place. Thus in the community setting, a shortage of GPs in inner city areas has led to experiments with an extended role for community nurses (Trnobranski, 1994).

With the implementation of the New Deal on junior doctor hours and the Calman proposals for the reform of postgraduate medical training (National Health Service Management Executive [NHSME], 1991g; Working Group on Specialist Medical Training, 1993), the amount of junior doctor time available for service provision has diminished. This has intensified pressure across all specialities for the emergence of new nursing roles which can absorb some of the work previously carried out by junior doctors be this clinical (for example venous blood sampling) or administrative (for example taking a patient history). Indeed, the Greenhalgh Report sponsored by the Department of Health (DoH) has recommended that a range of fairly basic junior doctor tasks should become part of the role of all registered nurses rather than simply added on post-registration (Greenhalgh and Co., 1994). Nursing's opposition to the 'off-loading' of relatively unskilled tasks generally echoes the sentiments of the Briggs Committee that:

> If the nursing and midwifery professions were to be expected to undertake a greater proportion of the more frequent, boring, inconvenient or time-consuming of the doctor's tasks, because of a false assessment of the similarities between the two professions, then the caring functions, to which we attach such basic importance, could be jeopardised. (Committee on Nursing, 1972: 47)

Where the proposed role development would lead to a more sophisticated practitioner there is no assumption that this also means more nurse autonomy but rather, parts of the nursing profession fears, more sophisticated forms of medically controlled training and delegation. For example, in 1994 Trent region's New Deal Taskforce introduced a nurse practitioner scheme encompassing 32 new nursing roles in 18 different Trusts in 16 specialties (Day, 1995; Hopkins, 1996). The scheme received a mixed response from the nursing profession which voiced the fear that if nurses become 'pseudo-medical assistants' or 'super-trained technicians' the traditional caring aspects of nursing would be lost to health care assistants (Read and Graves, 1994: 5).

This not an unreasonable fear. Much of the motivation behind the drive for a return to holistic nursing stemmed from the recognition that nurses are readily seduced by the medical–technical aspects of their work into seeing this as high status and basic nursing care as low status (Melia, 1987). To an extent this is a predictable problem. One proof of the existence of a medical hegemony in the Health Service is the automatic acceptance of a status hierarchy derived from medicine's knowledge base and the devaluation of other knowledge areas such as that of nursing. The medical profession has shown itself happy to encourage this process by providing the means for training and accrediting those nurses who aspire to take on aspects of doctors' work – for example, the role of surgeon's assistant accredited by the Royal College of Surgeons (Caine, 1993; Holmes, 1994). Furthermore, the ineluctable advance of ward-based medical technology can impact on the nurse–patient relationship in ways which inhibit the use of the holistic nursing approach (Wichowski, 1994).

The local innovations in practice associated with NDUs, primary nursing and nurse practitioners are seen by the nursing profession itself as part of what has become known as the 'New Nursing' movement. New Nursing is presented as assertively professional, as having broken with the 'handmaiden' legacy of nursing's past, and as autonomous of the medical hegemony (Salvage, 1992). In reality, we have seen how the practice innovations which are in the vanguard of the New Nursing search for empowerment are trapped in the embrace of medicine's dominance of the NHS workplace. To what extent have the policy initiatives pursued by the nursing profession suffered the same fate?

The policy challenge

From the early 1980s onwards, nursing's strategy has been to try to increase its professional power by gaining state support for policies which enhance the status of its self-regulating mechanisms in the areas of initial training and professional development and standards. Using policy sleight-of-hand, the state has responded by using the nursing profession's very ambition and, it has to be said, nursing's political incompetence as the vehicle for undermining nursing's power.

Initial training

Building on the principles of professional self-development enunciated by the Briggs Report of 1972 and the Judge Report of 1985 (Committee on Nursing, 1972; RCN, 1985), Project 2000 proposed that nurse education be reformed root and branch in terms of both content and delivery (UKCC, 1986a). A new curriculum armed with additional knowledge components would produce a new type of registered nurse who, in the familiar phrasing of the nursing process, would be 'able to marshall information, to make an assessment of need, devise a plan of care and implement, monitor and evaluate it' (UKCC, 1987: 5). With a sideways glance at the debate about holistic nursing and the degree of delegation which should occur therein, the nurse is described as a 'knowledgeable doer' who 'will be more actively involved in the delivery of care than at present' (*ibid.*). Schools of nursing were to be transferred from the restrictive (as it was seen) and service-dominated confines of the District Health Authority to the sunlit uplands of higher education where nurse students would study for their higher education diplomas and would become largely supernumerary with their service contribution reduced from 60 per cent to 20 per cent of their three year course (National Audit Office, 1992: 19).

The political ambition of the Project 2000 policy was to give nurse education the ability to establish an autonomous professional identity in high-status learning environments where the imperatives of medicine would no longer reign supreme. In fact, the profession has simply exposed itself to new pressures which, over time, are actually diminishing the control it has previously enjoyed in this field of self-regulation.

The fundamental power of any professional group is derived from its exclusive command of a particular knowledge territory. In this respect nursing has always suffered from its close proximity to medicine and its reliance on the knowledge of this more powerful neighbour. Up to the 1989 reforms of nurse training initiated in the wake of Project 2000, attempts to mark out nursing's own therapeutic field customarily focused on the carative–curative distinction with, at best, ambigous results. Hence the Briggs Report, for instance, noted that:

> all medical activities and developments affect nursing and midwifery directly or indirectly. We believe that while doctors, nurses and midwives are perma-

> nently partners in care, it is possible to distinguish in the first instance between the caring role of nurses and midwives (which involves coordination and continuity) and the diagnostic and curative functions of doctors: both have teaching and research functions. (Committee on Nursing, 1972: 44–5)

For nursing, the weakness of this distinction as a political device is that whilst medicine has a state-sponsored monopoly of cure, nursing competes with numerous other occupations for the title of 'the caring profession'. Traditionally, nursing's position within the medical hegemony had given it a protected status as a health care occupational group but as the profession pursued a therapeutic identity separate from, and a rival to, medicine this advantage rapidly diminished as nursing energetically sawed off the branch on which it had for decades sat.

The move into higher education has also provided the opportunity for nursing to give full reign to its self-destructive tendency to take other knowledge areas more seriously than its own, thus further diluting any claim it may have to being the proprietor of a unique knowledge field. Courses implementing the new Project 2000 curriculum have sought to integrate a variety of physical and social science components into a single nursing course in different ways in different institutions (Jowett *et al.*, 1994: 4). Students on the Common Foundation Programme (the first part of the course) have commented on the lack of course cohesion, the disjointedness, the difficulty of absorbing the breadth of the information generated by the range of subjects studied and their relief at commencing the Branch programmes with their more obvious nursing orientation (*ibid.*: Ch. 4). One commentary on the impact of this new approach on psychiatric nursing observed that:

> in striving to become a respected profession, psychiatric nursing is losing that unique body of knowledge and skills that defines it as a profession. Instead, the main emphasis seems to be on academic sociological and psychological principles, with little teaching of the practical skills of psychiatric nursing, which not only preserve a patient's dignity but also keep the patient alive. (Short, 1995: 303)

No longer directly subject to the service needs of the hospital, nurse education is now subject instead to the vagaries of the higher education institution and, lacking a core knowledge area, has assumed a range of new identities.

At the same time as displaying an unfortunate inclination to fragment its existing knowledge base and thus undermine its distinctive claim to the caring role, nursing has also failed to protect itself adequately against the emergence of competing claims from rival occupational groups. It was a government condition of state support for Project 2000 that a new breed of health care support worker should be created to compensate for the much reduced service commitment of nurse students. The UKCC accepted this condition, proposed that the new range of 'helpers' (as it called them) should be supervised by nurses and suggested that the UKCC and National Boards should 'have an important role in developing the helper concept, delineating roles and defining the instruction which may be required' (UKCC, 1987: 6). Wise words but, regrettably for nursing, not implemented. Unlike the medical profession, nursing failed to recognise that the colonisation of neighbouring occupational groups, and if necessary the judicious ceding of territory to such groups, is part and parcel of maintaining one's position in the occupational hierarchy.

Political pressure for a reassessment of the skill-mix between nurses and other carers in the NHS had, in any case, been present for some time and the new nurse training provided the opportunity for that pressure to become manifest. In 1986 the Committee of Public Accounts had reached the conclusion that there was significant scope within the NHS for the more efficient and effective deployment of nurses (National Audit Office, 1992: 16). The 1989 NHS Review echoed this theme and in *Working for Patients* determined that local managers 'will be expected to re-examine all areas of work to identify the most cost-effective use of professional skills' recognising that:

> This may involve a reappraisal of traditional patterns and practices. Examples include the extended role of nurses to cover specific duties normally undertaken by junior doctors in areas of high technology care and in casualty departments; the use of clerical rather than nursing staff in receptionist work; and making full use of midwives as recommended in the reports of the Maternity Services Advisory Committee. (DoH, 1989a: 15)

Considerable weight was added to this view by the 1991 Audit Commission report *The Virtue of Patients: Making the Best Use of Ward Nursing Resources* which showed that there was no consistent approach to setting ward establishments, that wide variations existed in the staff numbers on similar wards, that the staffing and skill-mix differences from day to day were greater than those between similar wards, and that analysis of the skill-mix data could find no explanation for the variations (Audit Commission, 1991: 27–44). However, the Audit Commission did find an explanation for the absence of an explanation when it observed that at the majority of hospitals change in the nursing service has been largely reactive. The report continued: 'It has not flowed from a clear idea about what nursing is, where it should be heading, or the structural changes needed to support its development' (*ibid.*: 58). So a random distribution of skill-mix is to be expected.

For a state preparing to invest in a new, and more expensive, form of nurse training this was not good news. As the National Audit Office pointed out, it meant that 'in the absence of comprehensive skill-mix reviews prior to introducing Project 2000 there is a risk that manpower forecasts and bids for funding may be based on existing staffing patterns which are inappropriate' (National Audit Office, 1992: 17). Furthermore, the state could reasonably ask, if the existing staffing patterns are inappropriate, what should they be? As there is no consensus on the appropriate methodology and criteria for assessing nursing workload (Bright, 1985; Buchan, 1992), this was at one and the same time an impossible question to answer and a political opportunity which the state could not afford to ignore.

Nursing and midwifery constitute 47 per cent of NHS expenditure on pay and since the early 1980s their costs have risen faster than any of the other NHS staffing groups (Audit Commission, 1991: 3). This is largely due to their success in getting the state to agree to the creation of a Pay Review Body and a system of clinical grading as well as the pay inflationary implications of Project 2000 and a more highly qualified nurse. In 1983, in due recognition of the RCN's steadfast maintenance of a 'no strike' policy, Prime Minister Margaret Thatcher established a Pay Review Body for nurses, midwives and professional technical and ancillary staff which, in terms of pay determination, placed nursing on an equal footing with the medical and dental professions. It also proved to be a useful vehicle for nursing to secure pay increases above the level of inflation. Also, in its fifth report in 1988 the Review Body recommended a new pay structure which would recognise the clinical expertise and responsibility held by clinical nurses. The cost of this new system of clinical grading was not only economic, with an overall increase of 15 per cent in expenditure on the nursing workforce (Hart, 1994: 225), but also political. Some 120 000 appeals were lodged against the grades initially awarded to nurses, with the result that lengthy and often acrimonious administrative frictions for a while became a feature of the local Health Service.

By the late 1980s the state had decided that nursing was a political nuisance to be dealt with: the size and cost of the nursing workforce continued to rise disproportionately to other sectors of NHS staffing, there was no known logic to the distribution of its skill-mix, nursing no longer recognised the medical leadership inherent in the concordat between medicine and the state, and it aggravated the doctors.

Project 2000 provided the state with the opportunity to diminish nursing's power because it was a nurse-led educational reform which destabilized both the profession's identity and the structure of its training system. It is surely no coincidence that at the same time as the schools of nursing were making their enforced transition from the NHS to higher education, the Nurses, Midwives and Health Visitors Act 1992 was downgrading the powers of the National Boards for nurse education and thus their ability to manage the process of educational change and protect the nursing interest. The Act removed the duty of National Boards 'to provide or arrange for others to provide education and training' and left them with the residual role of approving educational institutions and courses within the framework of UKCC standards (National Audit Office, 1992: 29). A year later in 1993, following the recommendations of Working Paper 10 of *Working for Patients* the Boards were stripped of their funding responsibility for nurse training and it was transferred instead to the Regional Health Authorities (DoH, 1989c). In future it was the Regions who, in consultation with consortia composed of representatives from employing Trusts, Health Authorities and GPs were expected to identify the demand for qualified nurses and decide on the number of students to be recruited and trained. In due course, these consortia became the budget holders and commissioners for nurse training with Regions acting as coordinators across consortia (NHSE, 1995d).

In a few short years, nursing lost control of the funding and key decision-making functions in nurse education. From a ring fenced budget, centrally allocated by a national professional body to a stable system of schools of nursing, nurse education moved to a regionally devolved budget, exposed to the attentions of rival occupational groups, with schools of nursing facing an uncertain and competitive future. The auguries are not favourable. Between 1986 and 1994 the numbers of nurse tutors fell from 8 200 to 6 570

(Hart, 1994: 245). More significantly, between 1987–88 and 1994–95 the numbers entering pre-registration education in the UK fell from 19 600 to 14 000 – a drop of 39 per cent – and the number of nurses qualifying fell from 37 000 in 1983 to 21 400 in 1995 (English National Board for Nursing, Midwifery and Health Visiting [ENB], 1995: 7; Seccombe and Smith, 1996). The effect of this has been an 11 per cent reduction in the entries to the UKCC register between 1989–90 and 1995–96 (Seccombe and Smith, 1996). Within nurse education itself, some schools of nursing have already closed and others have lost entire training contracts (Humphreys and Davis, 1995).

For the state, the necessary corollary of a reduction in the power and presence of nursing in the NHS is an increase in the numbers of support workers. Whether designated as 'nursing auxiliaries', 'health care assistants' or, more recently, 'generic care workers' this staffing group will be recruited from a wider ability pool than nursing, will require less time and finance to train, and will be less expensive to employ. The intention is that over time there will be a shift in the balance of skill-mix in the NHS workforce, with a lower proportion of registered nurses and a higher proportion of support workers (Buchan, 1992: 48). As could be expected from the discussion earlier, nursing is divided in its response to this development. On the one hand, the champions of undivided and personalised holistic nursing argue that the transfer of the less skilled tasks to support workers would undermine the therapeutic essence of nursing, dependent as this is on a close and continuous relationship between nurse and patient. On the other, the proponents of the skilled clinical nurse elite maintain that support workers provide nursing with the means better to manage the therapeutic relationship with the patient through the primary nursing approach (see for example Chief Nursing Officers for England, Wales, Scotland and Northern Ireland, 1993). The latter are quite happy to accept that the nursing profession will shrink in size, though not, they believe, in power, as a consequence.

Despite knowing that the support worker was an explicit condition of government backing for Project 2000, nursing has done little to ensure that the development of this rival occupational group occurred within its own sphere of influence. Support worker qualifications now form part of the NVQ system of competency-based accreditation which is designed to maximise flexibility of career movement within industrial and service sectors. Despite the good intentions of the UKCC quoted earlier, the input of nursing to the evolution and accreditation of the new support worker role within the NVQ care sector has been marginal. The UKCC could have offered its own NVQ-based certification and thereby given itself the power to define both the content of the support worker roles and their career linkages with the role of the registered nurse. Instead it has assumed the stance of the superior spectator and thus missed the chance of colonising this crucial piece of neighbouring occupational territory. The net effect is that as support workers gain qualifications and status so they are able to compete directly with nurses for provision of the less skilled care to patients. Given their lower cost, they have the advantage and Trusts are increasingly using skill-mix reviews as the means for adjusting the balance between the two groups in the support workers' favour.

Professional development and standards

It was nursing's intention that Project 2000 would form the basic building block of its bid for enhanced professional autonomy and power. But if the new Project 2000 nurses, armed with the nursing process, were to continue to assert their independence over a lifetime of professional activity in a workplace where the dominance of medicine was the norm, they would require the means for determining the direction of their own professional development. Traditionally, that direction had been determined locally within a set of procedures for the extension of the nurse's role which doctors controlled (DHSS, 1977). Within this procedure, nurses developed their role to the extent that doctors were prepared to delegate tasks. Post-registration qualifications issued by the National Boards were designed so as to facilitate this arrangement. Alternatively, registered nurses could opt for one of the specialist options and take a National Board course to become a midwife, health visitor or one of the several types of community nurses.

In 1992 this traditional system of hierarchical and certificated professional development accepting of the medical hegemony was replaced by one where the individual nurse's professional judgement became the single most important factor. In this year the UKCC issued its *Scope of Professional Practice* containing a list of principles which, it stated, should in future 'form the basis for any decisions relating to adjustments to the scope of practice' and 'should replace the system of certification for specific tasks' (UKCC, 1992:

12). At the same time, the long-established guidance on the extension of the nurse's role was withdrawn by a circular which stated baldly that 'each practitioner is personally accountable for their own practice and for the maintenance and development of their knowledge and competence' (NHSME, 1992). In future, stated the circular, decisions concerning professional practice should be based on the UKCC's *Scope of Professional Practice*, its *Code of Professional Conduct*, its *Exercising Accountability* and its Midwives Rules 1991 (*ibid.*, see UKCC, 1989, 1992a, b).

The clear objective of this radical shift of policy is the promotion of a model of individual professional autonomy directly parallel to that enjoyed by medicine. Instead of having their professional development structured by local procedures, doctors' preferences, and the views of senior nurse management, nurses would be free to determine their own professional destiny accountable only to the principles contained in the *Scope of Professional Practice*. It is an interesting ambition but, as with Project 2000, it both neglects the legal and political realities at the grassroots in the NHS and, in dismantling a proven system, exposes nursing to other pressures.

The *Scope of Professional Practice* did not make the legal position clear but it can be surmised that the *Code of Professional Conduct* and the law of negligence are the safeguards to ensure that the actions of individual nurses comply with those of a responsible and competent body of nurses, with or without a certificate (Hopkins, 1996: 36). With litigation for medical negligence on an ever-rising curve, Trusts are highly unlikely to be convinced by such vague assurances of correct professional behaviour and will continue to demand legally robust evidence that their employees are competent to practice before they are willing to take vicarious liability for nurses who have expanded their role. Merely because the medical profession has not dealt with this issue is no good reason, in the view of Trusts, to make the same mistake with nursing. To protect themselves, Trusts will require an agreement covering the expanded role to be made between the nurse and the employing organisation probably backed up by some form of certification of competence; an agreement which will almost certainly look remarkably similar to the old extended role procedure, because doctors will have to be included where delegation occurs.

In practice there is a large gap between the UKCC's assertion that nurses can now develop their professional identity simply through a personal dialogue with a list of principles, and the nature of medical power in the NHS. The law recognises this power. In their discussion of a case concerning a nurse's accountability for the delivery of treatment technically within the province of junior doctors, Dowling *et al.* conclude:

> The courts still appear to regard the relationship between doctor and nurse as one of professional and handmaiden where the doctor gives the orders and the nurse carries out the instructions. Such attitudes might influence a court to conclude that, *irrespective of the UKCC's professional nursing regulations*, the consultant is ultimately responsible for determining [the nurse's] competence and ensuring that she does not exceed it. (Dowling *et al.*, 1996: 1213, emphasis added)

Doctors therefore have a very real incentive to restrict the autonomy of nurses because this is what the law expects of them and the penalties for not doing so can be substantial.

What impact the implementation of the UKCC's new Post-Registration Education and Practice (PREP) policy will have on this situation it is difficult as yet to predict. Addressing the nurse the UKCC claims that PREP, introduced on 1 April 1995, 'radically changes the significance of your registration'. In future, it continues:

> your UKCC registration will not only mean that you have reached the necessary professional and academic standards for initial registration but also that you have, on a three-yearly basis, maintained and developed those standards through additional learning activities, for the benefit of patient and client care. (UKCC, 1995: Factsheet 1)

A direct parallel to the medical profession's emerging system of Continuing Medical Education (CME), PREP provides the means for the standards-linked monitoring of professional development. To retain their registration, nurses are required to undertake a minimum of five days of study, or its equivalent, every three years. Also, they can seek to attain the status of specialist or advanced practitioners. Specialist practitioners are required to take a National Board accredited course and if successful their new qualification is entered against their name on the UKCC register. This is clearly a device which enables the existing sub-groups within the profession to retain their identity and their old system of certification. Thus the eight categories of community nurse keep all the old distinctions intact (for example, district nurse, health visitor, community mental health nurse) (*ibid.*: Factsheet 6). Advanced practitioners, on the other hand, are a conceptual product of the new thinking associated with the *Scope of Professional Practice* in that they are seen as 'adjusting the boundaries for the development of future practice' and 'pioneering and developing new roles which are responsive to changing needs', as working at Masters and PhD level, but not (as yet) having their qualifications entered on the UKCC register (*ibid.*: Factsheet 7). It is emphasised that advanced practice is not an additional layer to be added to specialist practice.

In support of PREP, the English National Board for Nursing, Midwifery and Health Visiting (ENB) has introduced its *Framework for Continuing Professional Education and Higher Award for Nurses, Midwives and Health Visitors* (ENB, 1993). This provides nurses with a variety of 'links and ladders' with which to pursue their academic and professional development up to a Higher Award if they so wish. Although the *Framework* thus retains the principle of a hierarchy of certification in its implementation of PREP it does not couple certification with standards as the old extended role procedure had done. Having said that, however, it is noticeable that outside of the *Framework* the ENB is still developing courses to suit the specific requirements of the medical profession – for example, training for the nurse to act as assistant to the surgeon (*Nursing Times*, 1995) – and providing accreditation for the specialist practitioners, both of which do tie competence to certification. In practice, therefore, the ENB is running the old and new systems of professional development side by side and allowing nurses to choose the one they prefer. Neither is likely to enable nursing to enhance its professional autonomy because both are obliged to accept, either explicitly (the old system) or implicitly (the new system), the limits imposed by medical power.

In this respect, a key constraint on the professional development of nurses has always been the exclusive power of the doctor to prescribe drugs, restated in the Medicines Act 1968. According to the Act, a nurse may administer a prescription-only drug but only under the direction of a doctor. (The UKCC provides guidance on how this delegation should occur (UKCC, 1986b)). The Cumberledge report *Neighbourhood Nursing* recognised that the credibility of nursing as a therapeutic exercise would be considerably enhanced if nurses were given the power of prescribing, albeit for a limited list of drugs, and proposed such a reform as part of its advocacy of the nurse practitioner role in primary health care (DoH, 1986a: 33). Not surprisingly, the medical profession was decidely lukewarm about this idea since the right to prescribe presupposes the right to diagnose (or 'assess') the condition of a patient. Put the two rights together and you have a professional armed with the ability to challenge medicine's much coveted monopoly of the healing process. The Central Consultants and Specialists Committee (CCSC) made its reservations quite clear (Beecham, 1990), as did the community health doctors who were afraid it might lead to Health Authorities replacing them with less expensive nurses (Merry, 1990). In the event, the Medicinal Products (Prescription by Nurses) Act 1992 amended the Medicines Act to give a very limited set of prescribing rights to registered nurses with a district nursing or health visitor qualification who are employed by a Health Authority, Trust or Fundholding practice (Wright, 1996). Given that the employer is variously liable for the nurse's acts, it is also a requirement that such nurses undertake the appropriate training in order to protect the employer from negligence claims. Once again we see how the legal position inevitably leads to a version of the old extended role procedure regardless of what the *Scope of Professional Practice* may say. It is significant that nurse prescribing does not extend to nurses in hospitals, nor is such an extension envisaged.

In the final analysis, if nursing is to enhance its self-regulation in the sphere of professional development then it must exercise the dominant influence over the standards by which it is judged. In this respect, as in many others, nursing lacks the power to insist that its view should be the definitive one. Unlike medical audit, where the setting of standards is regarded as a matter for doctors alone, nursing audit is a field where the nursing profession has to compete with both doctors and managers for the final say, not only as to what standards are appropriate but also as to how the data collected in the course of nursing audit should be interpreted against those standards. Despite its attempts to use nurse quality assessment systems imported from the United States as a form of professional protection, nursing has had to accept that rival occupational groups consider that they have a legitimate input to make to any debate about nursing standards, not only through the filter of nursing's own data, but also in terms of other sources of information such as skill-mix reviews (Harrison and Pollitt, 1994: 105–11). The UKCC may happily assert that nursing has the exclusive right to monitor its own professional development but others with more power in the NHS such as managers will assert that this should instead be a shared responsibility and subject to corporate criteria.

It can be argued that midwives are excepted from the rule of management intervention and medical hegemony and that recent policy developments have reinforced their ability to act as autonomous professionals. In practice, it can be shown that their experience reflects the underlying reality faced by the rest of nursing. In 1992 the House of Commons Health Committee report *Maternity Services* concluded that the policy of encouraging all women to give birth in hospitals cannot be justified on the grounds of safety, that women should have a choice of maternity care and the option of home delivery, and that a 'medical model of care' should no longer drive the service (DoH, 1993c: 1). Pursuing the same line, the Expert Maternity Group's *Changing Childbirth* report recommended that:

> Every woman should be given the name of an individual midwife who works locally, to whom she can go for advice and help throughout her pregnancy. In many instances this named midwife will also be the lead professional – undertaking the key role in the planning and provision of care. (*ibid.*: 5)

Midwives, it would seem, are being given unequivocal state support for their role as independent practitioners. It is, however, a role which is contingent upon the pregnancy being defined as 'uncomplicated'. Only a doctor through a medical examination and diagnosis can legally determine whether or not a pregnancy is uncomplicated and this decision occurs at the initial assessment of the pregnant woman. The midwife's right to care for the patient is therefore conditional upon the doctor's decision and, effectively, delegation has occurred. Thereafter, the midwife's autonomy is further circumscribed by rule 40 of part V of the Nurses, Midwives and Health Visitor Rules 1983 which imposes an obligation on the midwife 'to seek assistance from a registered medical practitioner where there is an emergency or where the midwife detects a deviation from the norm in the health of the mother' (*ibid.*: 39). It is in the weave of such rule systems that the fabric of medical power reveals its existence.

Conclusions

Nursing's traditional role in the politics of change in the NHS was to provide the appropriate support to the concordat between medicine and the state. Doctors controlled the demand for health care through their diagnostic function and nursing helped deliver the required treatment. In exchange for their acceptance of the medical hegemony, nursing got protection. The profession was given clinical autonomy at the ward level within medically defined limits, day-to-day control over the disposal of ward resources (a limited form of political autonomy), and economic security from the day they registered as qualified nurses in that Health Authorities guaranteed them a position following training. Further rewards came with the system of professional self-management for nurses implemented following the Salmon Report which, in many ways, was the high point of nursing power in the NHS: nursing was easily the largest occupational group in the Health Service, it had a sound hierarchical system of professional accountability and control, and it accepted the basic tenets of medical dominance.

Like other colonies, nursing chose to bid for independence and, in so doing, may well prove to have sowed the seeds of its own destruction as a force in the NHS (Salter and Snee, 1997). Ironically, the challenge was modelled upon certain characteristics of the medical profession which, nursing assumed, would if transferred give it the elixir of professional autonomy. In particular, the erroneous assumption was made that if nursing acquired an autonomy based on the individualistic nature of medicine's professionalism, it would simultaneously have gained an equivalent mantle of power. What nursing failed to comprehend was that this individualism is powerful because it is rooted in, and recognised by, the adminstrative apparatus of the Health Service with the full support of the state. Nursing has no such recognition and so any assertion of autonomy on its part remains simply that: an assertion.

Its strategy for achieving the intended state of professional autonomy encompassed the establishment of nursing as a therapy in its own right, the creation of a distinctive knowledge area, changes in nursing practice, and the wholesale reform of nursing's education and professional development systems.

The attempts to test the claim that nursing can have a therapeutic effect independently of the medical input centred on the Nurse Development Units (NDUs) but these experiments were inconclusive and always subject to the limits of medical tolerance. They did nonetheless act as vehicles for the refinement of the nursing process, the method for the assessment and treatment of the patient which nursing has used as its professional alternative to medicine's diagnosis-based procedures. Originally imported from the United States, the nursing process has been the principal conceptual framework from which much of the subsequent practice and educational developments have taken their lead. Nurse practitioners have claimed that it enables them to deal appropriately with unscreened patients and primary nurses that it is a suitable tool for the management of patients at ward level. Both claims have aroused the opposition of doctors because they threaten to disrupt medicine's ability to determine what patients are treated where and for how long – in other words, patient demand.

Project 2000 also embodied the nursing process in its curriculum design and intended that the translation of nurse education from the NHS to higher education would facilitate the training of a new type of nurse able to think and act independently. This may well be the case. Unfortunately for nursing the move has also resulted in a curriculum with a fragmented knowledge base which overlaps with that of other caring occupations and dilutes any claim regarding the uniqueness of nursing's therapeutic contribution. Equally importantly, the state has used the opportunity afforded by the reform of nurse education to diminish nursing's power in this area of its self-regulation. The National Boards have suffered a diminution of their regulatory functions and the funding of nurse education has been devolved from the Boards to the regional and sub-regional level with a consequent loss of professional protection for the budget. Furthermore, as a condition of its backing for Project 2000, the state gained nursing's acquiescence in the creation of a new group of carers, the support worker, which, given its lower training and employment costs, is now a significant occupational rival which nursing has failed to control.

Pursuing the logic of the self-directive professional, nursing has reformed its post-basic system of professional development and standards monitoring through the introduction of the *Scope of Professional Practice* supported by new arrangements for Post-Registration Education and Practice (PREP) and a more flexible certification programme from the National Boards. Yet the legal position of the nurse and the reality of medical power at the local level remained unchanged. The result is a dichotomy between the conception of the autonomous nurse professional enunciated by nursing's national bodies and the actuality of life in the hegemonic order of medicine which embraces the NHS.

Having chosen to step outside the magic circle of medical protection and seek its own destiny, nursing is beginning to have to count the cost of freedom. With the minimum of ceremony, the Griffiths reforms removed the gains in nurse self-management associated with the Salmon Report and substituted the general management structure of accountability which views nursing as just another occupation to be managed for the corporate good (DHSS, 1983a). In its ever-intensifying search for efficiency and effectiveness general management has exposed nursing, as the largest single element in the NHS cost base, to continuing pressure from which there is no longer any escape. Gone are the days when nursing could rely on the institutional inertia of the NHS bureaucracy to protect it from such pressure and it has sufficiently alienated the medical profession to ensure that there will be little support from that direction. Having increased their unit costs through more expensive training, a more highly qualified workforce, an aggressive Pay Review Body, and an inflationary system of clinical grading, nurses have priced themselves out of a job. The same self-destructive urge has seen them ignore the implications of the emergence of the rival support worker, fail to colonise its certification system, and thus acquiesce in the undermining of their own occupational position. In practical terms this has meant that fewer nurses are being trained and entering the register, that they are no longer guaranteed a post on completion of training and that contractually they are more insecure (Stock *et al.*, 1994): clear evidence of professional decline.

The search for a new professional identity based on the individual nurse has served to fragment the traditional forms of nursing influence founded as they were on national, hierarchical arrangements. The declining power of nursing's national training bodies has been emphasised by the continuing frictions and rivalries between nursing's two main unions: the RCN and Unison. Faced with the inevitable reduction in the number of qualified nurses, these organisations are bound to compete and thus ensure that nursing is unable to mobilise the principal political strength of its mass membership.

As for potential allies, neither medicine, managers nor the state have an interest in maintaining a high cost and ambitious occupation as the numerically dominant element in the NHS workforce. Having opted for decolonisation but with the concordat between medicine and the state alive and well, nursing may well have to accept that its survival now depends on its reaching a fresh accommodation with medicine based on its clinical and management expertise.

7

Community Care

Introduction

For the most part, the politics of change in the NHS can be understood purely in terms of health policy issues. The Health Service was founded on the assumption that it should have a national rather than a local or regional identity, it has vertical lines of management accountability to the National Health Service Executive (NHSE) and the Department of Health (DoH), its funding is nationally determined and dispensed, and in general it acts as a discrete political structure.

Community care policy challenges both the idea and the substance of this separateness and, in so doing, provides a distinctive input to the dynamic of change at work in the NHS. In analysing the path and effect of this contribution, this chapter deals first with the additional social rights incorporated within the various mutations of the community care concept, their relationship with health care rights, and the nature of the composite political demand thus produced. Second, it explores how the logic (or non-logic) of the community care policy requires health and social care agencies to control or redirect the demands upon them. Third, the reverse of the coin, it examines how that same logic encourages agencies fiercely to protect the supply of resources at their disposal. Finally, given the tension between the inevitability of the demand–supply mismatch, the imperatives of agency accountability and the interests of the power groups involved, the chapter traces the strange distortions imposed on the detail of policy implementation.

Origins of the policy

As the Social Services Committee observed in 1985, 'the phrase "community care" means little by itself' and has 'come to have such general reference as to be virtually meaningless'. Instead, the Committee continued, 'it has become a slogan with all the weakness that that implies' (Social Services Committee of the House of Commons, 1985: x). But having documented the numerous and different usages of the term from care by families and volunteers rather than statutory care, through the transfer of responsibility from the NHS to Local Authorities, to the pursuit of the ideal of normalisation, the Committee was obliged to recognise that, slogan or not, it was here to stay and had to be addressed as a policy issue. Although undoubtedly epistemologically correct, the Committee was missing the political point: the power of the term 'community care' derives precisely from the fact that it does not have a specific meaning but is a powerful political symbol within the pantheon of the welfare state, used by many to legitimise fresh additions to the list of state protected social rights. Interestingly, the Committee added its own weight to that process when it defined community care thus:

> Appropriate care should be provided for individuals in such a way as to enable them to lead as normal an existence as possible *given their particular disabilities* and to minimise disruption of life within their community. (*ibid.*, emphasis added)

The phrase 'given their particular disabilities' is the only limitation imposed on the otherwise universal application of the social rights contained in this definition and would present few problems to the inventive lobbyist.

In the context of the original Beveridge conception of the welfare state as founded upon the pillars of education, health and social security, the ideological significance of the development of community care policy, in whatever manifestation, is that it has progressively eroded the barriers between the three policy areas, encouraged cross-fertilisation between the different types of social rights embedded in each and created political pressure for the expansion of existing rights or the creation of new ones. Of the three areas, health was the only one to offer an absolute and unconditional social right, universally applicable to the whole population and which aimed for the optimum quality of service. The 1946 National Health Service

Act made it the responsibility of the Secretary of State 'to promote the establishment of a comprehensive health service' available free and from the cradle to the grave. By way of contrast, the 1944 Education Act made the social right of education contingent upon age, the 1946 National Insurance Act made the right to pensions, sickness and unemployment benefits contingent upon contributions, and the 1948 National Assistance Act made the right to national assistance contingent upon a 'means-test' and pegged it at the minimum, subsistence level. In retrospect the key ideological question for the welfare state was whether those social rights with a contingent status of one kind or another would acquire the absolute status of the social right to health care. Once this happened, a fresh impetus would be added to the spiral of political demand which any party of government would find difficult to handle.

From the beginning, not only were the three policy areas less than watertight but, more significantly, there was in any case a not very well hidden fourth area, which today is called 'social care', with considerable growth potential. Both the 1946 NHS Act and the 1948 National Assistance Act contained provisions which gave Local Authorities certain duties and powers to develop what was effectively a social care function, though the structure of the legislation shows clearly that in the *ad hoc* tradition of welfare growth these were, at the time, seen as largely unrelated provisions. The NHS Act allowed Local Authorities to employ home helps, gave general discretionary powers for the care and aftercare of persons suffering from illness and for preventive measures relating to health (paras 28–9). More categorically, the National Assistance Act enlarged the social rights of particular groups. First, it gave Local Authorities the duty to provide welfare services for those of its residents who were 'blind, deaf or dumb, and other persons who are substantially and permanently handicapped by illness, injury or congenital deformity or such other disabilities as may be prescribed by the Minister' (section 29). Second, it laid a duty on Local Authorities to make accommodation available for all persons who by reason of age, infirmity or any other circumstances were in need of attention not otherwise available to them (Part III, section 21). Interestingly, only the provisions of the NHS legislation allowed Local Authorities to charge for their service.

By giving Local Authorities the responsibility for fulfilling the right of selected groups to different types of social care, but by providing no logic to the process, the state randomly scattered the seeds from which the versatile plant of community care was to flourish. The hidden fourth pillar of the welfare state was in place and the next 50 years were to see an elaborate scaffolding of client groups and caring services erected around it. As each new group was admitted to the fold of social care rights, the critical political question was whether it was given absolute or contingent rights. On the answer to this question rested the ability of the state to control and, if necessary, limit the extent of its responsibility for the demands expressed by these groups.

The first two groups to receive a clear extension of their rights into the social care field were the mentally ill and the mentally handicapped. In 1957 the Royal Commission on the Law Relating to Mental Illness and Mental Deficiency argued for care for 'mentally disordered patients with no more restriction of liberty or legal formality than is applied to people who need care because of other types of illness' and that this should be supplied as non-institutionalised care by Local Authorities (Royal Commission on the Law Relating to Mental Illness and Mental Deficiency, 1957: 3–4). Because this was a case of absolute health care rights being directly transposed to the embryonic sphere of social care there was never any question that in that sphere they should be expressed in contingent form, regardless of how difficult it might be to meet absolute social care rights in practice. The Commission's recommendations were duly given legal status in the Mental Health Act 1959.

But for two further groups, the elderly and the disabled, the acquisition of social care rights was less clear cut. For the elderly, the Health Services and Public Health Act 1968 was the first post-war legislation to enhance the social care rights they already possessed under the National Assistance Act. Local Authorities were given powers to provide home helps, visiting, and social work and warden services. However, the exercise of these powers remained discretionary, the social care rights of the elderly were contingent upon that discretion and charging for services was permissible. Similarly, for the disabled, although the Chronically Sick and Disabled Persons Act 1970 placed a duty on Local Authorities to provide a service, this provision was contingent upon the needs identified by the Local Authority and the resources it had available. Again, charges could be levied for the services provided.

Although, to a greater and lesser degree, health and social care rights for the mentally ill, mentally handicapped, elderly and disabled had thus been merged at the statutory level, no parallel change had been promoted at the level of service delivery in order to ensure the implementation of these rights. By 1970 the ideological shift towards a more comprehensive welfare state with an expanded concept of citizenship rights broadly using the rhetoric of 'community care' was well established but the policy and bureaucratic separation of health and social care remained intact. Within Local Authorities the organisation of the growing social care functions had been characterised as 'piecemeal and haphazard' by the Seebohm Report *Local Authority and Allied Personal Social Services* and order was sought through the creation of a single social services department in each authority (Seebohm Report, 1968: para 309). But operational integration across the NHS and local authority divide remained negligible despite the continuing ideological pressure from government policy documents such as *Better Services for the Mentally Handicapped* (DHSS, 1971) and *Better Services for the Mentally Ill* (DHSS, 1975).

By the early 1980s the absolute social right to health care had been carried across the NHS–Local Authority boundary by these four client groups and taken root as rights to social care contingent upon such factors as Local Authority resources and policies and client income. But because for two decades this process had been labelled 'community care', and as 'individual needs assessment' had by now entered the lexicon of community care language, the point was inevitably reached where restricting social care rights to the members of four client groups came to seem illogical. Why should they be so privileged given that health care is available to all? Furthermore, if health care rights are abolute, why should social care rights be contingent?

In the light of these two questions, and the range of new political demands they represent, official documents of the 1980s on community care make interesting reading. The development of welfare state values had reached the point where they had, *pace* the New Right, boxed in the politicians. The *ad hoc* growth of social rights had produced a *de facto* and incremental policy of community care which glaringly lacked any infrastructure to implement it. On the other hand, treating community care as a distinct policy area in order to facilitate the necessary policy implementation would be to create a natural political forum within which additional claims for social rights could be happily, and logically, registered.

The difficulty of restricting the groups to whom community care is applicable, that is making community care rights non-universal, when discussing the policy in the public domain is apparent in the DHSS's 1981 document *Care in Action*. This refers to community care for the main client groups of 'the elderly, mentally ill, mentally handicapped, disabled people *and children – as well as for the special and smaller groups such as alcoholics*' (DHSS, 1981: 7, emphasis added). The Audit Commission's *Making a Reality of Community Care* (1986) echoes this definition and the Griffith's Report *Community Care: An Agenda for Action* plumps for the four priority groups and the catch-all of 'similar groups' (Griffiths, 1988: 3). By the time the White Paper *Caring for People* was published in 1989, community care had moved a long way from its specific client group origins. The four main client groups may provide the structure for the document but the universal applicability of community care rights is not denied. As it points out, 'Many people need some extra help and support at some stage in their lives, as a result of illness or temporary disability' and, in particular, 'People with drug and alcohol related disorders, people with multiple handicaps and people with progressive illnesses such as AIDS or multiple sclerosis may also need community care at some time' (DoH, 1989f: 10).

As the rights embodied in the official definitions of community care have become progressively more universal, and hence more akin to health care rights, so the pressure has grown to give them absolute status as well and so remove the long-standing distinction between health care and social care rights. From the mid-1980s onward, added pressure in this direction also came from the social security arm of the welfare state as official recognition was made of its contribution to community care. In its 1986 report the Audit Commission commented that 'social security payments have played a major part in promoting care in the community' (Audit Commission, 1986: 43). It identified three benefits most relevant to meeting the cost of caring for the ill and disabled: attendance allowance, invalid care allowance and supplementary benefit payments for board and lodging (independent homes). Although these three rights to social care were, and are, conferred as the result of professional assessment, once given, only the supplementary benefit payment is contingent upon a means-test. Furthermore, and this is of critical importance, unlike the rights to health care and Local Authority social care, social security rights are not delivered by a state structure with a fixed budget. Traditionally, they have constituted an open-ended entitlement with no expectation that they should be constrained by the availability of state finance.

Controlling demand

The continuing expansion of rights to social care, supported and encouraged by the broad ideological commitment of all political parties to the welfare state, by the cross-fertilisation of universal and absolute rights from health and social security to the Local Authority sector, by the adaptability and power of the slogan of community care, and by the legislative recognition enshrined in the NHS and Community Care Act 1990, now confronts the reality of the limits to welfare imposed by a tax base which has expanded more slowly than the demands placed upon it, combined with the reluctance of taxpayers to increase the proportion of their income which they give to the state. Given the rate of increase in the costs of community care, it was always going to be a difficult policy area to bring under control.

Using a broad definition of community care which included health, social security and Local Authority components, the Audit Commission calculated that in the ten years up to 1989–90 publicly funded community care had increased 70 per cent in real terms from £8.45 billion to £14.3 billion (1989–90 prices): a rate of increase which meant that whereas in 1979–80 the community care budget had equalled that of the NHS hospital budget, by 1989–90 it was 40 per cent higher (Audit Commission, 1992b: 3). Adopting another measure, *Caring for People* notes that gross current expenditure on 'core community care services' rose from £1169 million in 1979–80 to £3444 million in 1987–88 – a real terms increase of 68 per cent (DoH, 1989f: 3). Within this, social security support for people in independent residential care and nursing homes rose from £10 million in 1979 to over £1000 million in 1989 (*ibid.*); by 1993 the figure had risen to £2575 million (Health Committee of the House of Commons, 1995b: vii).

Having given its citizens an array of community care rights, the state faces the problem of how to control the rapidly rising demand and cost associated with them. Its position is complicated by the fact that any attempt to limit citizenship rights to community care necessarily challenges the hegemony of the welfare state values and the belief that social rights should be increased but not reduced. As yet, the hegemony prevents the public (though not private) recognition by the state of the choices it faces and the covert policy of control being pursued. The effect is to create a paradox within government policy on community care which the parliamentary Health Committee has summarised as follows:

> the paradox at the heart of the new policy which all participants must seek to resolve is that the new arrangements will operate within the two parameters of cash limits and assessments of need. One side of the equation aims to restrain what has been in the past an open-ended commitment to people claiming Income Support, whilst the other is intended to identify levels of need as never revealed before. This is likely to produce a contradiction between downward pressure on budgets and increasing demand. (Health Committee of the House of Commons, 1993: 42)

The resolution of the contradiction is essentially an exercise in the selective allocation of resources, or rationing – a normal enough political task except when the ideological context is adamantly opposed to it, as it is here. Unable to confront the problem at the national level the state has delegated it to the Local Authorities which, as the lead bodies for the implementation of the 1990 legislation on community care that came into effect on 1 April 1993, have the interesting task of imposing cash limits in a policy field previously accustomed to a considerable subsidy from the largesse of social security funds. In so doing, they are expected and obliged to act in collaboration with other agencies and in particular with the NHS.

Regardless of the rhetoric of cooperation which pervades the community care field, it remains a structural fact that each contributing agency is accountable for its budgeting decisions to quite different masters and that officers are formally responsible for protecting the integrity of their budgets. To the extent that they fail to control the demands upon these budgets, the agencies' officers will be held culpable. Given the requirements of accountability and the sanctions for failing to meet them, it is therefore in their interest to maximise their agencies' power over the way in which the demand for community care is defined and channelled. This is particularly critical in the case of the NHS because if the demand is not dealt with, redirected or nullified its final destination is always going to be the accident and emergency department of the local hospital.

Within much of community care, 'needs assessment' is the formally approved method for determining whether an individual, or groups of individuals, can exercise a particular social right and therefore place a demand upon the community care agencies. Much in vogue at present, the assessment of the need for care, either for an individual or a population, is presumed to be undertaken by a professional who decides what care is required using the criteria peculiar to that profession. Naturally enough, criteria will vary both within and between professions and will produce the kind of inter-professional disputes which we have already seen associated with the purchasing function in the NHS (see Chapter 2). Whichever professional group (and here we are talking about doctors, nurses and social workers) wins such a dispute will also win the power to control access to, and hence demand for, community care – a significant power from the point of view of both those citizens wishing to exercise their social rights and the health and social care agencies who will be asked to arrange the care deemed necessary.

Making social rights contingent upon professional judgement is not a new idea. Making such contingency explicit, however, is. The right to health care, for example, no matter how absolute the surrounding rhetoric may have made it sound, was in practice always contingent upon the medical judgement (needs assessment) of GPs and consultants. Within the community care policy, this hidden contingency is promoted to the level of public principle and then linked to a further limiting factor: that of available resources. Thus *Caring for People* points out that:

> Assessments will therefore have to be made against a background of stated objectives and priorities determined by the local authority. Decisions on service provision will have to take account of what is available and affordable. (DoH, 1989f: 20)

It then becomes the responsibility of the Local Authority to make public their criteria of eligibility for assessment and the way in which their assessment processes will work (*ibid.*). Commenting on the impact of eligibility criteria, the Audit Commission observed, perhaps optimistically:

> Authority members and senior managers who previously determined service levels and allowed staff locally to ration services, will in future need to take the decisions about rationing, leaving service decisions to commissioners. This turnabout places rationing decisions firmly where they should be – with politicians and senior management. (Audit Commission, 1992b: 26)

Unfortunately, putting rationing decisions where they should be, wherever that is, will not necessarily render them legitimate so far as the general populace is concerned, because explicit rationing will inevitably be seen as a further constraint on the social rights once so freely given.

Nowhere is this more obvious than in the case of the elderly who found their rights to community care radically trimmed under the

1990 legislation as a result of the transfer of responsibility for the provision of their residential and nursing-home care from the open-ended social security budget to the cash-limited budgets of Local Authorities. Whereas previously the elderly had enjoyed an unrestricted entitlement to private (but not public sector) residential and nursing-home care through the payment of Income Support following an amendment to the Social Security Act in 1982, from 1 April 1993 this absolute right was ended and potential elderly clients were to be assessed by the Social Services Department of their Local Authority. The effect of this was that suddenly their rights became contingent upon the Local Authority resources available.

Making rights and assessment procedures dependent upon the resources available may control demand (assuming they are used to do so), but it will also offend the values of care management which increasingly permeate the social services field. Care management and assessment are a set of officially sponsored procedures deemed to 'constitute the core business of arranging care which underpins all other elements of community care' (Department of Health [DoH], Social Services Inspectorate and Scottish Office Social Work Services Group, 1991: 7). Originally advocated by the Griffiths Report *Community Care: An Agenda for Action*, care management aims to:

> identify and assess individual's needs, taking full account of personal preferences (and those of informal carers), and design packages of care best suited to enable the consumer to live as normal a life as possible. (Griffiths, 1988: 1)

It is a method which, according to DoH guidance, 'makes the needs and wishes of users and carers central to the caring process' (DoH *et al.*, 1991: 16), promotes 'the rationale for this reorganisation [which] is the empowerment of users and carers' (*ibid.*: 11), and 'gives users and carers a more powerful voice in expressing needs and influencing the services they receive' (*ibid.*: 55). Although these kinds of statements are duly balanced by appropriate genuflections to priority setting and rationing (*ibid.*: 45–6), it is clear that the ethos of care management equally lends itself to generating, as much as controlling, the demand for community care.

Within the overall demand equation, a key question is whether the need identified is a health care need or a social care need since on this decision rests the allocation of the demand either to a health care purchaser (Health Authority, GP Fundholder) or to a social care purchaser (Social Services Department). (Also, from the client's point of view, if the need requires social care then the Social Services Department may charge for its delivery whereas health care is always free.) Very wisely in the light of its strategy of avoiding the political flak associated with the implementation of the community care policy, the DoH made it clear that there would be no national definition of the health–social care demarkation and devolved the problem to the local level. Given the nebulous nature of community care, it was inevitable that there would be numerous fraught negotiations between local agencies in an attempt to resolve the health versus social care issue and hence determine who had to do what. Initial advice from government served only to emphasise the metaphysical quality of the definitional discussion and the difficulty of distinguishing between a citizen's rights to health and social care (DoH *et al.*, 1991: 85–6).

The NHS and Community Care Act 1990 gave Local Authorities not only the lead responsibility in community care but also the formal duty of bringing apparent health care needs to the attention of the appropriate Health Authority (section 47). Technically, therefore, they hold the initiative in developing assessment procedures and the definitions of health and social care which are needed to underpin these procedures. This is particularly important in the case of the elderly, the largest and fastest growing client group in community care, where there is a clear incentive, if not imperative, for Local Authorities to use their control of assessment as a mechanism for ensuring a match between the demand for social care and the budget which became available to them as a result of the transfer of monies from social security via the Special Transitional Grant (STG) – regardless of the implications for the other agencies. *Caring for People* made it plain that 'the new funding arrangements for residential care mean that discharged hospital patients will have to undergo assessment of their care needs before the "care" costs of residential accommodation can be met at public expense' (DoH, 1989f: 49). By implication, elderly patients are not to be discharged until the Local Authority has agreed to meet the social care costs thus incurred. Bearing in mind that Local Authorities can legitimately adjust their assessment criteria to suit the resources they have available, where these resources are limited they may refuse to agree to discharge, thus producing blocked beds in hospitals and an unreleased pressure of demand. This situation may be reinforced by the patients themselves who may wish to avoid early discharge to residential or nursing homes where they face means-tested charges

(Thornicroft *et al.*, 1993: 770). Before the 1990 legislation there was an incentive for hospitals to discharge their patients into such homes knowing that the patients' social security rights would ensure that the state met the social care costs thus incurred. This option is no longer available.

Alternatively, Local Authority decisions to place elderly people in residential and nursing homes, rather than leave them in long-stay hospital beds, could create new demand for the community health services: GPs and community nurses. Again, the early signs following the introduction of the new community care policy were that this was in fact happening. In its report *Priorities for Community Care* the British Medical Association (BMA) noted with concern that an increase in residential and nursing homes means an increased workload for GPs because the residents are registered individually with GPs. In some areas the numbers of such homes are so high that they may account for up to 80 per cent of GP visits (BMA, 1992: 25). Then there was the further question of how this redirected demand would impact on the NHS purchasers, particularly given the acquisition by GP fundholders in April 1993 of the community health services (community nursing) budget for their patients with the balance being retained by the Health Authorities. In this situation the response to uncontrolled Local Authority-created demands upon NHS resources was always likely to be both fragmented and lukewarm. Fundholding practices would regard their new obligation to buy community nursing services as a disincentive to press for the early discharge of their patients from hospital (Thornicroft *et al.*, 1993: 770).

On the other side of the coin, in the case of the client groups of people with a learning disability and the mentally ill, the closure of institutions has resulted in the transfer of individuals into the community where their social care is now the responsibility of the Local Luthority, without a corresponding transfer of finance from the Health Authority (Audit Commission, 1992b: 10; BMA, 1992: 25).

Inter-agency disputes about who should pay for what service are an inevitable consequence of devolving the control of demand issue to the local level, yet to begin with the new policy recognised neither the possibility nor the consequences of such disputes. As the Royal College of General Practitioners (RCGP) has pointed out prior to the implementation of the new policy:

> Where different professionals, or authorities, have different opinions with regard to what care is required there is no mention about any mechanism which will exist to deal with such a situation. If the Social Services Department and Health Authority disagree about what is required for a patient, neither the patient, relatives, nor GP... have any right of appeal. (RCGP, 1992: para 7.1; see also Browning, 1992: 1416)

Originally, conflict resolution was not part of the policy of community care because, formally, conflict of interest between the different agencies was assumed not to exist. Instead, the language of joint assessment, joint planning, joint working and, occasionally, joint commissioning was used as a universal panacea for all the policy's potential ills sucessfully obscuring any sensible analysis of the points of political tension and any discussion of how they might be managed. However, once the policy was launched, the joint Regional Health Authority (RHA) and Social Services Inspectorate (SSI) monitoring of the policy's implementation recognised the emerging difficulties and required Health and Local Authorities to put arbitration procedures into place.

Nonetheless, the dominant official view was that community care plans would facilitate the inter-agency collaboration required to make the community care policy work and, thereby, prevent local conflicts. How realistic was this assumption? The 1990 NHS Act and subsequent policy guidance gave Local Authorities the responsibility for producing community care plans on an annual basis. In so doing they were to consult with Health Authorities who were also obliged to produce plans setting out their community care policies. Wherever possible, both authorities 'should take a joint approach to planning and ensure their plans are complementary' and 'at an early stage' agree 'on the key issues of who does what, for whom, when, at what cost and who pays' (DoH, 1990c: paras 2.3, 2.11 and 2.12).

Such ambition deserves to be rewarded but the initial evidence was that the majority of community care plans amounted to position statements rather than strategic documents which sought to commit specified resources to particular objectives (Wistow *et al.*, 1993). Indeed, as early as 1992, monitoring by the RHAs and SSI revealed 20 out of the 108 Local Authorities 'floundering' in producing their plans (Moore, 1992b: 12). This merely confirmed the experience of three decades of attempts to create local power-sharing through central exhortation. The 1962 Health and Welfare Plans, the 1970s Local Authority Personal Social Services (LAPSS) plans, and joint planning from the mid-1970s onwards, all foundered on the elementary political fact that the agencies involved had different lines of accountability and no incentive to cooperate (Hardy *et al.*, 1990; Hudson, 1992). Why community care plans should be expected to confound this historical experience is unknown. Instead, there was every likelihood that they would be an annual paper exercise which satisfied the statutory requirement but had no impact on the underlying political issue of joint management of the demand for community care (Salter and Salter, 1993).

Protecting supply

If the first political imperative of local health and social care agencies is to seek to control the demand placed upon them, the second is to protect their ability to meet the demand. Retaining control over key areas of funding and decision-making will allow an agency to limit the effects of excess demand upon its service, protect its supply of that service and hence render it less vulnerable to charges that it has failed to implement its part of the community care policy. In the absence of centrally imposed mechanisms of demand control, reinforced by joint lines of accountability and equal penalties for overspending, agencies will seek to maximise their power over resources and their allocation.

In a global sense, their ability to do so is circumscribed by the size of the national cake available and the way in which it is sliced up. In this respect it is the Local Authorities who are most exposed because they are taking on fresh responsibilities with only limited information on the increased costs thus incurred and no guarantee that central allocative procedures will adjust Local Authority budgets to meet the new costs. In the case of the elderly client group, a key question for Local Authorities was what money was to be transferred to them from the social security budget over what period. Hence it comes as no surprise to learn of the tensions within the 'Algebra Group', which had the job of developing the national transfer formula, between the Local Authorities' Association (LAA) and the DoH (Health Committee of the House of Commons, 1993: 6–7). Formula setting is a highly political exercise and the LAA argued that the formula proposed for determining the Special Transitional Grant (STG), as it was known, would leave them £289 million short of funds for community care in 1993–94 (*ibid.*: 18). Equally as important as the absolute size of the community care budget for the elderly is the protection, or lack of it, that it will be afforded within a Local Authority's overall allocation via the Revenue Support Grant (RSG). As a ringfencing mechanism, the STG operated only for a four-year period and was phased out in 1996–97. Thereafter, the transferred funds were subsumed within the Personal Social Services Standard Spending Assessment baseline and distributed through the RSG, at which point the ringfencing and protection of this community care budget came to an end. The issue then became one of how far Social Services Departments within Local Authorities were able to ensure that their budgets actually reflected the amounts notionally allocated by the DoH for community care.

The Griffiths Report recommended a ringfenced budget for community care for both Health Authorities and Local Authorities as a necessary requirement of policy implementation (Griffiths, 1988: 17–18). Although Health Authorities do not have a ringfenced budget as such, they do have established patterns of expenditure on the four main client groups of community care and, given the political will (admittedly a large caveat) have a framework which can be used to maintain that overall level of spending within the new purchasing arrangements. What they have no incentive to do is to transfer what they regard as a protected budget to the Local Authority arena, where it will almost certainly immediately become relatively unprotected. As a protection of supply issue, this is most clearly apparent in the case of the dowry system.

In 1983 the DHSS circular 'Health and Service Development: Care in the Community and Joint Finance' (HC[83]96) set up the dowry system for the mentally ill and people with learning disabilities, whereby a Health Authority would transfer funds to a Local Authority for each patient resettled from a long-stay institution into the community. As a system for rechannelling finance, it was slow in taking off. Audit Commission research showed that in 1989 60 per cent of Health Authorities had still to reach agreement on the financial and practical arrangements for resettlement. Of those who had, considerable difficulties had been encountered in negotiating the dowries, with the result that they were often inadequate or not paid in perpetuity (Audit Commission, 1989, quoted in BMA, 1992: 19). More recent evidence suggests that the situation has been rendered more complex by the post-1991 purchaser–provider division which has severely tested the limitations of the original 1983 guidance. In Bath, for example, the transfer of monies for the social care of 400 people with learning disabilities required agreements to be concluded between the Health Authority and two County Councils, between the Bath Mental Health Care Trust and the Health Authority, between the Trust and the Counties' Social Services Departments, and between the Trust and the voluntary agencies providing accommodation for clients (Dobson, 1992).

The Audit Commission has rightly pointed out that:

> any agreement between agencies for one authority to assume a changed responsibility for a particular area of activity in the community cannot easily be reflected by any change in the finance allocated to that authority from the centre. These difficulties are a direct feature of the way central government determines and distributes finance. It is not ideally suited to fund policies that require constant adjustment at the margin between different authorities. (Audit Commission, 1992b: 11)

Recognising this problem, Griffiths proposed that the Local Authorities should at least have the certainty of a centrally allocated specific grant released on approval of their community care care plans (Griffiths, 1988: vi). This would have given their Social Services Departments the confidence to plan their services on the basis of predictable budgets and, equally important, would have reassured Health Authorities that their transferred funds could be attached to a stable purchasing core. The clear disadvantage of such an arrangement from the national political perspective, however, is that it would have given the DoH and ministers an unwelcome visibility when the budgets proved inadequate to meet demand and would have severely compromised their strategy of making rationing a local issue.

Periodic pleas for the joint commissioning of community care by Health and Local Authorities as a mechanism for overcoming budget protectionism ignore both legal and political realities. It is by no means clear how the legal restrictions on the use of Health Authority finance for social care and Local Authority finance for health care could be dealt with in order to make consortia arrangements work effectively (Audit Commission, 1992b: 23). It remains the simple, but frequently ignored, fact that 'as long as services are funded through discrete routes and controlled by separate bodies with different priorities and accountabilities, this goal [of joint commissioning] is likely to be difficult to attain' (Audit Commission, 1992a: 35). There is no incentive, and potentially large penalties, for such common-law marriages.

Given that resources are finite, the imperative to protect supply must also apply to decision-making about the delivery of service. If Health and Local Authorities were in some sense compatible when understood in terms of geography, method of resource allocation, expenditure on client groups, culture, and history of integrated working, then there would be a general basis for the negotiation of shared areas of decision-making. The evidence suggests the opposite is true. Before the District Health Authority (DHA) and Family Health Service Authority (FHSA) mergers of 1996, only about a quarter of DHAs related geographically to Social Service Departments on a one-to-one basis and in some places DHA and Social Service Department boundaries were 'hopelessly entangled' (Audit Commission, 1992b: 12). There was no correlation between DHA spending on community health services and expenditure by FHSAs and Social Service Departments on related services (*ibid.*: 14). Nor was there any evidence of a substitution effect between acute, community health service, GP and social service provision – that is, they are not complementary services (Audit Commission, 1992a: 12). Finally, there was very little joint provision and that which did exist was poorly coordinated (*ibid.*: 19).

In the absence of shared assumptions about appropriate levels and patterns of provision, the abrogation of decision-making power is an irrational act because it is difficult, if not impossible, to predict the consequences of such a move. Attempts to construct models of inter-agency decision-making in community care, usually underpinned by a benign and non-political belief in the cooperative intentions of all concerned, have served only to emphasise the daunting complexity of such relationships and the imaginative abilities of certain government agencies when asked to help with implementing non-implementable policies (DoH *et al.*, 1991: 58; Audit Commission, 1992a: 35, 1992b: 30, 1992c: 59). Even if the Health and Local Authorities could agree a realignment of decision-making powers, they would still have to persuade their respective professionals (doctors, nurses, social workers, care managers) that the new lines of authority and accountability thus established made professional as well as managerial sense.

For most professions, particularly medicine, relinquishing territory to another professional group is a difficult step to take. In some cases they may be legally prevented from doing so. Consultant community psychiatrists, for example, are responsible for the discharge and aftercare of their patients under the Mental Health Act

1983 and difficulties have arisen in integrating their decisions with the care management approach of the Social Services Department (see for example Thornicroft *et al.*, 1993: 771). GPs, meanwhile, are contractually independent and fiercely resistant to any encroachment on their territory as a result of the community care policy (RCGP, 1992). In other cases, the new policy may require a profession to give up some of its professional power and hence its ability to protect its service resources. It is significant that in its evidence to the Health Committee, the Association of Directors of Social Services (ADSS) expressed concern that whereas hospital consultants want a swift assessment and discharge of their patients (typically within 48–72 hours) in order to reduce waiting lists, Social Services care managers with the responsibility for making the assessment for discharge to social care may want two weeks to carry it out (Dobson, 1993). Consultants want to retain control to prevent the blocking of beds, maintain throughput and fulfill contracts, and care managers want to implement fully the new discharge policy. The agenda, responsibilities, and accountability lines of the two professional groups are different and the road to a negotiated solution a rocky one (Smith, 1993).

Policy implementation

The analysis thus far has explored the political implications of the community care policy for the agencies involved at the point at which the policy was implemented in April 1993 (see Salter, 1994a). It is of course possible that this analysis has overestimated the significance of inter-agency and professional divisions and jealousies and understimated the will of central government to drive through the implementation of the new arrangements, insist on inter-agency cooperation, invent common systems of accountability, impose procedures for the resolution of boundary disputes, bang professional heads together, and confront the demand–supply mismatch in welfare. Mindful of that possibility, this section investigates the implementation of the 1990 community care legislation and assesses its implications for the NHS.

One of the principal community care policy objectives is 'to provide a service in which the boundaries between primary health care, secondary health care and social care do not form barriers seen from the perspective of the service user' (DoH, 1990c: 5) –

implying a centrally driven programme of organisational change. From the beginning, however, there was no indication that the central authorities really wanted to shift from a stance of policy implementation through exhortation, to one where the penalties for non-implementation of community care were greater than the instinct of local agencies for self-preservation through non-compliance and the maintenance of their separate identities. To do so would have brought the DoH into the front line of policy accountability. Indeed, it was more prudent for the Department to give direct responsibility for the implementation of the new policy to the local agencies and for itself to retain the more distant, and safer, role of provider of encouragement and support.

In pursuance of this low profile approach, implementation circulars were issued stating what should be done (notably the 'Foster–Laming' letters of 11 March and 25 September 1992 with a checklist of eight key tasks – EL[92]13 and EL[92]65), a joint RHA–SSI monitoring programme was initiated to check on progress and disseminate good practice, and the DoH-based Community Care Support Force offering much rational advice appeared in the lead up to April 1993 (see for example Community Care Support Force, 1992). But within this supportive net there was very little that had to be done on pain of 'something worse than nurse'. Community care plans had to be produced, and four of the Foster–Laming 'eight key tasks' were included in Regions' corporate contracts with DHAs, but there is no evidence of sanctions being applied for their non-fulfillment. Only in the case of discharge arrangments for hospital patients requiring social care, which had to be in place by 31 December 1992, was a financial sanction applied: if Local Authorities did not have discharge policies agreed with the relevant Health Authorities they would not receive their Special Transitional Grant. This condition was then retained and tied to each subsequent annual allocation of the STG during its four-year life; though how effective a policy control this constituted was, as we shall see shortly, questionable.

Given that most of the implementation advice and monitoring criteria focused on service systems and managerial criteria, it was perfectly possible for the implementation process to be judged a success by the DoH, as indeed it was so judged, even though there was little change experienced by service users and carers (Henwood and Wistow, 1995: 25). Such an approach to policy implementation, where organisational processes are elevated above policy outcomes, has led one informed observer to describe community care as 'just a fairy tale' (Warner, 1995).

But as the organisational complexities of achieving the utopia of a seamless service of community care have become ever more apparent, so the fairy tale has become less believable. Given the range of groups involved and their manifold care requirements, full implementation of the policy's ambitions effectively demands joint working between every agency of the welfare state. Taking the example of the mentally ill, the Audit Commission noted that the government 'needs to reaffirm its commitment to comprehensive local services and to coordinate the responsibilities of the Departments of Health, Environment, Education, Employment, Social Security, and the Home Office' – apparently unaware that this is administratively impossible (Audit Commission, 1994c: 8). At a more focused level, Hudson has ably demonstrated the numerous bureaucratic impediments to integrating the provision of community accommodation by Housing Departments with the procedures of the NHS and those of Social Security : assessment methods are separate and different, funding criteria inconsistent, and inter-agency understanding limited or non-existent (Hudson, 1996; see also Goss and Kent, 1995).

As the fiction of inter-agency cooperation has become threadbare and as the initial policy implementation measures have run their course, so the state has found its strategy of distancing itself from the policy's effects difficult to sustain: being 50 miles behind the front line is of little use when the front line has dissolved. Except for the initial tranche of implementation measures, the only permanent mechanism for achieving inter-agency collaboration has been the community care plan (CCP), and central support for this has been lukewarm. New guidance on CCPs was issued to Local Authorities in 1995 but this was non-directive and only served to broaden the function of the plans and so further dilute their impact: CCPs were to act as a source of accountability to local residents, a vehicle for purchasing strategies and provider business plans, and a means of meeting central and regional monitoring requirements (DoH and Department of the Environment [DoE], 1995). No new incentives were provided to encourage policy implementation and there was every likelihood that official exhortation to work jointly would, as Hudson observes, 'be met with marginal and cosmetic changes to an already inadequate cosmetic relationship' (Hudson, 1995a: 238; see also Hudson, 1995b). To add insult to injury, parallel guidance created a new potential area of demand on health and social care agencies by insisting that CCPs should be integrated with local Community Care Charters with their inevitable lists of new social rights (DoH and DoE, 1994).

With hindsight it is clear that it was only a question of time before the local tensions between agencies tasked with implementing an over-ambitious and poorly supported policy would surface at the national level. Two client groups in particular have ensured the national visibility of the limitations of community care: the elderly and the mentally ill. In both instances the key issues have been the control of demand and the protection of supply.

For ten years the open-ended Department of Social Security support for the elderly in residential and nursing homes had absorbed and obscured the growth in the demand for continuing care, to the cost advantage of both Health and Local Authorities. Between 1982 and 1993 the number of residents supported by Social Security rose from 16 000 to 281 000 (Health Committee of the House of Commons, 1995b: vii). During the same period the number of Local Authority Part III residential home places fell from 116 000 to 69 000 and between 1976 and 1994 the number of NHS beds specifically designated for elderly people fell by one-third from 55 000 to 37 000 (*ibid.*). The use of beds also changed: between 1989 and 1994 the throughput in the geriatric service of the NHS increased by more than 60 per cent and the average length of stay reduced by a third (Wistow, 1995: 25). Demand from the elderly for health and social care was being re-directed using a loophole in the system which also allowed the Health and Local Authorities to reduce their financial commitment to this politically weak client group, protect their available resources, and ignore the consequences. Well before the implementation of the 1990 community care legislation, the effect of this administrative sleight-of-hand was already apparent in terms of the health care needs of those in residential homes. A 1990 survey showed that the majority had progressive diseases requiring medication, 20 per cent of whom had not been seen by their GP since admission (Grosney and Tallis, 1991: 32).

The community care policy introduced in 1993 closed the loophole and diverted the demand back once again to the Health and Local Authorities – much to their chagrin, as over the previous decade they had grown accustomed to the social security subsidy and duly re-allocated their elderly care budgets to deal with other, more pressing, matters. Theoretically, the STG was supposed to meet the supply-side implications of this sudden re-routing of demand, but in practice it did not. As the pressure mounted upon the Local Authorities' budgets (now formally responsible for the provision of nursing and residential home places for the elderly) their response was to raise the political visibility of the issue; delay acceptance of the demand in order to protect their supply base; and try to re-direct at least some of the demand through the negotiation of agreements with the NHS concerning the boundaries between health and social care.

By November 1994 a quarter of all Social Services Departments (SSDs) were reported as having insufficient money in their STGs to maintain their purchasing patterns to the end of the financial year (Wistow, 1995: 25). At the same time the reluctance or inability of SSDs to assess elderly hospital patients for discharge to community care in a timescale which suited the hospitals led to the blocking of beds. A survey by the NHSE in March 1995 found that of all patients aged 75 and over occupying a hospital bed 20 per cent were waiting to be discharged and of these a third were awaiting placement in a residential or nursing home (Health Committee of the House of Commons, 1995b: xxiii). In the same year a British Medical Association (BMA) survey found that 82 per cent of geriatricians reported that the new assessment arrangements delayed the discharge of medically fit patients, with the average number of extra days thus spent in a bed being 17 (BMA, 1995b). Bedblocking in turn had a knock-on effect on the ability of Trusts to deliver their contracts: 45 per cent of Health Authorities in 1995 gave bedblocking as the reason for the failure of their Trusts to meet their service provision targets (National Association of Health Authorities and Trusts, 1995). The inevitable point had been reached where officers of local agencies became rather more interested in survival than they were in cooperation.

Enter the DoH. With the definition and management of the boundaries between health and social care now the key issue for local agencies faced with the enhanced demand from the elderly client group, and with the House of Commons Health Committee lending its weight to the prominence of the issue at the national level, the Department was obliged to abandon its arms-length approach to policy implementation. Yet it was reluctant to be too precise regarding the criteria which should be used to determine an individual's eligibility for free long-term health care as opposed to means-tested social care since this would defeat the devolutionary intent of the community care policy. As the Health Committee observed, 'the question of the precise administrative level within the NHS at which eligibility criteria are set can thus be seen to be essentially a political question' and recommended that there should be a 'nationally set framework' (Health Committee of the House of Commons, 1995b: xviii).

The Department duly obliged and produced the circular *NHS Responsibilities for Meeting Continuing Care Needs* which set out 'a national framework of conditions which all Health Authorities must meet in drawing up local policies and eligibility criteria for continuing health care and in deciding the appropriate balance for services required to meet local needs' (DoH, 1995e: 1). As political fudges go this document is a masterpiece because it is essentially promulgating criteria about criteria: specifying the range of continuing care services which should be provided, the discharge procedures and eligibility policies which should be in place, and the annual monitoring arrangements which will be used to ensure compliance. In effect it is enunciating criteria about organisational arrangements but not dealing with the detail of the criteria which these arrangements should then seek to establish in order to differentiate between health and social care. Had the Department done so it would have been publicly trapped by the collision between the absolute rights of the Health Service and the contingent rights of social care, and duly pulped. As a subsequent survey of the draft local policies and eligibility criteria produced by English Health Authorities in response to this circular showed, the criteria are capable of widely different interpretations according to the levels of resources available locally. Only a third of Health Authorities drew explicit boundaries of responsibility between themselves and the corresponding Local Authorities. Furthermore, the policies are not transparent in terms of patients being able to understand them, rarely incorporate objective and reproducible measures of dependency, and leave the ultimate decision to the clinician. The authors conclude, 'A harsh critic might say that what [the circular] and most of the surveyed draft policies and eligibility criteria say is that you are entitled to NHS continuing care if a doctor says you are' (Saper and Laing, 1995: 23). As this is the principle upon which the entire NHS is founded, and the natural resort of the DoH official under pressure, one should not perhaps be too surprised by this finding.

The Local Authority side of the health and social care divide is a mirror image of the NHS experience. Here there have been equally inconclusive attempts to develop eligibility criteria as the means for husbanding limited resources. Different definitions of 'dependency', 'risk' and 'need' have been used in different ways to establish different priorities amid what the Audit Commission has described as 'a maze of different criteria' (Audit Commission, 1996b: 14). Inevitably the consequence has been a wide variation in access to services accompanied by a range of different charging policies (*ibid.*: 31).

By using constructive ambiguity as a management art form, the Department has sought to create the illusion of positive central action whilst re-directing political attention back to the local level where boundary disputes between health and social care agencies will continue to be part and parcel of official life. However, the tactic of bouncing the responsibility for the demand from the elderly back and forth between Health and Local Authorities has had a knock-on effect on primary care which may well cause the issue to surface once again at the national level. The DoH itself recognised that the new arrangements could have considerable implications for the GP's gatekeeper role:

> Whereas previously they [GPs] were able to arrange admission directly to residential care or a nursing home for patients eligible for social security support, under the new arrangements GPs have to refer the person concerned to the social service department for a formal assessment. This in turn could have implications for GPs and primary health care teams if more people in vulnerable circumstances remain at home whilst awaiting assessment and placement and fewer are admitted to residential or nursing homes following the asessment of their needs. (DoH, 1994c)

The evidence is that these fears were justified. A 1995 BMA survey of general practitioners revealed that 54 per cent of GPs felt their workload had increased as a result of the community care reforms. Of these, 85 per cent said it was due to their having more dependent patients at home. At the same time, Local Authority services were seen to have deteriorated: home helps (by 65 per cent of GPs) and admissions to residential care (45 per cent) and nursing homes (39 per cent) (BMA, 1995a). How long before GPs decide that these pressures must cross the threshold of political visibility is an interesting question.

One answer is that it will not be long if the demand from the mentally ill continues to rise at its present rate in the face of numerous difficulties with the implementation of community care for this client group. Even in 1991 a third of practices surveyed in South West Thames Region said that the discharge of mentally ill patients had unduly affected their workload (Kendrick *et al.*, 1991). Since then the demand on the community services has increased, stimulated not only by the reduction in hospital beds for the mentally ill (down from 150 000 in the mid-1950s to under 43 000 in 1996) but also by the introduction of community mental health teams (CMHTs) which have opened up the service to a new range of clients with less severe illness and by schemes to divert patients away from the courts and prisons (Ford and Sathyamoorthy, 1996; Woodhead, 1996). Meanwhile, the odd, if not perverse, incentives unintentionally contained within the community care policy have encouraged the recognition of certain types of demand whilst sidelining others.

GP Fundholders, who since 1993 have had a budget and a responsibility to provide care for the mentally ill in the community, have focused on the largest client group: the less severely ill. They have a financial incentive to send the most severely mentally ill to a hospital's accident and emergency department to avoid paying for a domiciliary visit by a qualified Community Psychiatric Nurse (CPN), reinforced by a professional doubt about their own ability to deal with a client group of which they have little experience (Hadley, 1996). The difficulties faced by CMHTs and GPs in accepting the demand from the severely mentally ill has diverted it back to the hospital sector where the supply of beds is being reduced. The combined effect of these pressures is then registered in terms of high admission thresholds, wards where over 50 per cent of the patients are detained under the Mental Health Act and spillover into the high cost private sector. A one-day bed census of 12 inner London mental health services carried out in June 1995 revealed an average of between five and six patients per service in private psychiatric hospitals at any one time (Woodhead, 1996: 26).

Keeping these pressures off the national political agenda has been rendered impossible by a series of well-publicised homicides and suicides by psychiatric patients. Following *The Report of the Inquiry into the Care and Treatment of Christopher Clunis* and continuing public concern over the issue, the Department of Health was obliged to introduce fresh guidance on the discharge of mentally disordered people and their continuing care in the community; supervision registers were duly introduced in April 1994. As political firefighting goes, these measures provided the Department with some relief and allowed it time to produce more considered guidance to try and protect itself from the national heat generated by its policy failure. Following the style adopted in the case of continuing care, this took the form in *Spectrum of Care* (whimsically and non-threateningly issued under the Health of the Nation initiative) of a list of local services which should be provided for people with mental health problems (DoH, 1996a). The key problem of how these disparate services should be coordinated was then addressed in *Building Bridges* where, following long-established custom, heartfelt pleas were made for joint agency working, in this case among Health Authorities, GP Fundholders, Social Service Departments, Housing Departments, primary health care teams, specialist psychiatric services, community mental health teams, the voluntary sector, the independent sector, the criminal justice system, users, relatives and carers (DoH, 1996b: 25).

For reasons discussed earlier in this chapter, it is doubtful whether such exhortations have, or are meant to have, anything other than a symbolic significance (though such symbolism may be politically significant in that it disguises the intransigent problems of policy implementation in this field). As the Audit Commission sadly observed in its review of mental health services in 1994, 'apart from a few exceptional individuals, there has been nobody in a position to drive the changes through, despite widespread agreement with the policy' (Audit Commission, 1994c: 8). This is because it is in no-one's interest to drive it. For the policy to be implemented there would have to be a transfer of funds from the Health Service to Local Authorities, yet the pressures on Health Authorities documented above render them extremely reluctant to undermine their own supply base by giving away money. The size of the resulting implementation problem can be gauged from the distribution in 1992–93 of the total £1.8 billion budget for adult mental health services in England and Wales. Most of it was spent in the NHS (two-thirds of this on in-patient care) with only £185 million allocated to Local Authorities including a Mental Illness Specific Grant (MISG) of £31 million (*ibid.*: 6). Small wonder then that mental health care was traditionally a low priority for many Local Authorities. To change the balance of this expenditure, in the absence of a coordinating agency with statutory powers to iron out the inevitable local squabbles, is to risk political self-immolation and no-one is about to try it.

If single-agency responsibility were introduced for the health and social care of the mentally ill (as has been suggested by the Green

Paper *Developing Partnerships in Mental Health* – DoH, 1997) it would have to confront the further implementation problem presented by the disparate and frequently antagonistic professional groups involved in the delivery of that care. Three approaches in caring for the mentally ill are currently in use: the Care Programme Approach of the NHS – described by the DoH as 'the cornerstone of the Government's mental health policy' (DoH, 1996b: 45), the procedures embodied in section 117 of the Mental Health Act 1983, and the care management approach used by Social Services Departments. These approaches are based on different professional assumptions and protocols, have different lines of accountability and create manifold confusions in the way in which the care is actually delivered (Mental Health Foundation, 1994). Coordinating systems of management are non-existent with the result that the community mental health team, for example, has been described by the Audit Commission as 'a loose collection of independent professionals with freedom to decide what they do, when, and with whom' (Audit Commission, 1994c: 41). Even within a single agency, therefore, professional fragmentation would remain a significant obstacle.

Conclusions

The NHS and Community Care Act 1990 provided a fresh basis for the statutory relationship between the NHS and other agencies and hence a complex new input to the dynamic of change in the Health Service. Local Authorities were given the lead responsibility for the implementation of the community care policy and Health Authorities were required to work with them. It was intended that in the place of the long history of fudged relationships in the delivery of health and social care would come order, sweetness and light. But, as the Audit Commission has pointed out, the joint change agenda confronting the agencies was a very large one:

> They must identify needs more systematically; policy formation must become more clearly defined and overt, and must be shared between authorities; operational arrangements for commissioning care must be aligned with delegation of authority where appropriate, with budgets to match; and a host of other adjustments must be made to assessment procedures, service agreements, information systems, quality control and to the management of individual services. (Audit Commission, 1992b: 22)

In the historical context of proven difficulties of joint working between the agencies concerned, a touching reliance on goodwill and cooperation, few additional resources, separate lines of accountability, and only very limited and easily avoided sanctions for non-implementation of the policy, managing change on this scale was always going to be a tall order – particularly given the continuing demands on the service generated by the hegemony of welfare state values.

The hegemony insists that citizens' rights should be maintained or increased but not reduced and is impervious to the corresponding cost to the state of its expanding duties. In the case of community care, the impact of the hegemony is complicated by the historic difference between the citizen's absolute right to free health care, his/her contingent right to means-tested social care, and the pressure for the two types of rights to be merged with an inevitable increase in demand. Whilst part of social care was funded through the open-ended social security budget, the rising curve of social care demand was obscured. With the removal of that safety-valve by the ending of Income Support for the elderly in private residential and nursing accommodation in 1993 and, to a lesser extent, the demise of the Independent Living Fund for the severely disabled in 1992 (Hudson: 1993), the demand then had to be contained within a cash-limited Local Authority budget.

Local agencies are therefore faced with both a massive change agenda and an intensified rationing function. In order to ensure some kind of match between the demand for community care and the resources available, Health and Local Authorities must seek to maximise their individual powers over assessment and access mechanisms (demand control) and the supply of services. Separate budgetary accountability prevents them from doing otherwise. So whereas the formal change agenda of community care requires agencies to dissolve barriers and act collaboratively, the informal rationing agenda created by a state unable to accept the necessity of public limits to welfare rights, requires them to retrench, protect and husband their separate resources. Indeed, the Audit Commission has observed that there is a perverse incentive for the unilateral withdrawal of service by an agency in the hope that the other agency will have to pick up the provision and thereby save it money (Audit Commission, 1992c: 56).

Self-protective action must in turn produce innumerable local tensions and disputes between the purchasers and providers of health and social care as each seeks to pursue the policy of community care whilst limiting the political damage to themselves. Each fresh negotiation of eligibility criteria redefines the boundary between health and social care and creates a different input to the Health Service. Each failure to negotiate a settlement means that the problem is formally delegated to the professionals who make the decisions about assessment and access. Even where eligibility criteria are agreed, they are frequently sufficiently obscure to require interpretation by professionals anyway and thus, given finite resources, act as a focus for inter-professional disputes around the control of the rationing function. Consultants, GPs and nurses vie with social workers and care managers for the power to determine which patients should go where and who should pay for them. Within the NHS, other tensions arise between primary and secondary care, between GPs and consultants, in the struggle to determine who should deal with the health component of community care. But ultimately, it is always the medical profession which patrols and maintains the Health Service boundaries.

At the national level, the state is prevented by the hegemony of welfare state values from dealing directly with the demand for community care since this would entail an explicit reduction in community care rights. Nor is it particularly happy to advise Health or Local Authorities on supply side problems if this means being seen to take national responsibility for who gets what. Yet the scale and visibility of the policy implementation problems have forced two client groups, the elderly and the mentally ill, on to the national agenda so that the Department of Health has been forced to issue guidance. In so doing, the DoH has inevitably erred on the side of caution in its avoidance of statements which are too prescriptive and too specific, as such statements could all too readily generate criteria by which the success or failure of the guidance could be measured. How long it can use administrative ambiguity to disguise the impact of the demand–supply mismatch in community care is an open question.

For the time being the Department has no alternative. The political pressure for the expansion of community care rights continues unabated. For example, following its success with its proposals on the Community Care Charter, the Health Committee of the House of Commons has proposed that there should be a Long Term Care Charter which specifies the minimum levels of provision that people can expect Health and Local Authorities to provide (Health

Committee of the House of Commons, 1995b: xx). And in the same report the Committee notes that as a result of another of its recommendations carers have gained the statutory right under the Carers (Recognition and Services) Act 1995 to have their individual needs assessed by their Local Authorities (*ibid.*: vi). The state-sponsored encouragement of further demand continues.

Attempts to redirect the demand for community care to the private sector through proposals such as those contained in *A New Partnership for Care in Old Age* are unlikely to meet with much success in the short term given the present political culture and various technical difficulties (Chancellor of the Exchequer *et al.*, 1996). As yet only a small minority of people expect to have to pay towards care in their old age (Hudson, 1995c). There is also a large degree of actuarial uncertainty around the calculation of risks in old age, insurance premiums are high and as a consequence only 10 000 policies were estimated to have been taken out by the end of 1994 (*ibid.*).

For the NHS, therefore, there will be a continuing need to defend its borders, husband its resources and limit the effects of the community care policy on its internal dynamics. Whilst in general the Health Service can rely on the medical profession to continue to carry out its defensive role, the situation has been complicated by the perverse incentives inherent in the GP Fundholders' capacity to purchase community health services. As is customary, it falls to the Health Authorities to manage the resulting tensions between primary and secondary care.

8

The Private Sector

Introduction

As the demand on the welfare state continues to increase while the supply of tax revenues reaches its electorally acceptable limit, the state faces some key political choices. Should it seek to control or redirect the demand for welfare? Should it seek to achieve a better match between the demand for welfare and the supply of tax revenues through a more efficient use of existing resources? Or, finally, should it find ways of combining the supply of tax revenues with alternative funding mechanisms?

Whichever choice, or combination of choices, the state makes will inevitably involve a review of its relationship with the non-public sector of private finance and private provision. Nowhere is this more apparent than in the National Health Service where the continuing imbalance in the demand–supply equation, despite real increases in the NHS budget, is a constant source of political tension and will remain so regardless of which party is in office. Although there have for many years been objective political pressures for an examination of the relationship between the social rights which fuel the demand for welfare and the limits to the state's ability to supply it, and although such an examination would logically have to include the changing position of the private sector as an alternative source of welfare supply, social policy theorists have studiously failed to confront this issue. No framework has emerged to explain the dynamic which shapes the private–public sector relationship and to inform the choices which the state is now obliged to make.

The purpose of this chapter is to develop such a framework using the theoretical perspective on the politics of welfare established in Chapter 1. The chapter begins with a review of the existing social policy approaches to the relationship between the private sector and the NHS, identifies the assumptions and confusions therein and advances an alternative perspective. Second, it examines the various definitions of the private sector and their implications for any state-sponsored change in the frontiers between the private sector and the NHS. Third, it analyses the risk and accountability issues faced by the state in its political management of the private–public relationship in general and the Private Finance Initiative (PFI) in particular.

Perspectives on the private sector and NHS relationship

Traditionally, much of British social policy theory as been strongly influenced by the gently socialist values of its Fabian ancestry. Within this tradition, public services have an icon status and the private sector is represented as the purveyor of inequality, social division and privilege. Titmuss in particular argued that public administration is both qualitatively different from, and morally superior to, management in the private sector because it does not involve profit making, has to be concerned about human needs, and is more strictly bound by ethical codes of behaviour than the self-interested and wayward manager in the private market (Pinker, 1992: 280). Duly armed with this normative perspective, it is not entirely surprising that later writers in the genre have construed their primary analytical task as one of uncovering any threats to the welfare service from the private sector enemy, reflecting on the inequalities such changes will inevitably produce and constructing ways of countering such calamities. Cause and effect are thus in a sense dealt with, but in a teleological form which guarantees a particular conclusion. This is certainly true of those dealing with the way the NHS has related to the private sector.

Indeed, such is the opprobrium in which the private sector is held that some feel obliged to present their credentials as upholders of the NHS and socialized medicine. Thus in what has become a standard text on private health care, *The Business of Medicine*, Higgins emphasises that she 'began this book because of a deep commitment to the fundamental principle upon which the NHS was based' and that 'the real debate… is whether Britain has become "less socialist" as other countries of Western Europe have become "more socialist" and… whether the NHS is now "socialist" enough'

(Higgins, 1988: 3). Similarly, Mohan concludes a thoughtful article on private medical care with a sudden call to arms: 'Campaigns for socialized, and against commercial, medicine have to tackle this issue head on and seek not only to remove the concessions given to the private sector but to reverse the Tories' public expenditure priorities'. For without such an alternative social strategy, he continues, 'the Thatcherite welfare state could win by default' (Mohan, 1986: 359).

In the context of such values, the causal sequence is regarded as unproblematic: an all-powerful Conservative government (the natural enemy), strongly influenced by the ideas issuing from New Right think-tanks such as the Institute of Economic Affairs (IEA) and Adam Smith Institute (ASI), enacted policies which supported the private sector and undermined the NHS, with a resulting increase in social inequality (see for example Mohan, 1986, 1992; Papadakis and Taylor-Gooby, 1987; Taylor-Gooby and Lawson, 1993). There are, nonetheless, some differences of opinion regarding the forces driving this causal sequence. Papadakis and Taylor-Gooby take a functionalist approach and argue that the purpose of privatisation is to sustain the structure of class and gender advantage already present in the welfare state and to increase the gap between the middle mass and the marginal groups 'at the bottom of the pile' (Papadakis and Taylor-Gooby, 1987: 38–9). Within this perspective, the Conservative government and its policies are presented as pawns in a larger functionalist game. Mohan, meanwhile, is rather more inclined to ascribe causal primacy to a rational and skilful Conservative government encouraged and inspired by the all-pervasive ideas of the New Right (Mohan, 1992: 39–41). Interestingly, in his later work with Lawson, Taylor-Gooby not only adopts this latter view but develops it further. After listing the possible explanations of the use of markets in welfare delivery (for example social change, the limits of static bureaucracies, consumerism, changes in information technology) they decide that:

> The changes must be understood in their context as policies pursued by a particular government and crucially affected by its ideology and its conception of its own electoral interests. New technology provided an opportunity. Determination to cut spending demanded that the opportunity be grasped in a particular way. *Economic crisis, social change and public choice arguments provide convenient justification for change*. (Taylor-Gooby and Lawson, 1993: 146, emphasis added)

Such was the psephological sophistication of the Conservatives, it is claimed, that their welfare policies were intended to buttress their political advantage through the selective identification and treatment of their electoral supporters (*ibid.*: 143). Even Mohan is reluctant to see the Conservatives as quite so adroitly manipulative as this interpretation suggests and instead emphasises the constraints imposed on the Conservative government by the long-standing support among voters for the NHS (Mohan, 1986: 341).

The Fabian socialist perspective on the private sector–NHS relationship is such as to exclude analyses which do not share its belief both in the inherent superiority of state services and in the malign intent and power of the Conservative party to undermine them. Welfare pluralists, of whatever shade, have always been regarded suspiciously despite their common commitment to the welfare goal of social justice. Like the Fabian socialists, welfare pluralists are essentially advocates of a particular form of welfare delivery: they start with a belief in the inherent virtues of, say, the voluntary sector and then construct arguments to justify it. Unlike the Fabian socialists, however, they maintain that the provider role of the state should be limited and that the state should act principally as an enabler and regulator of non-state forms of provision (see for example Hadley and Hatch, 1981; Hatch and Mocroft, 1983; Brenton, 1985). Underpinning this view is a belief in the need to revise concepts of social justice by upgrading rights to risk and diversity at the expense of the traditional emphasis on security and equality (Evers, 1993: 11). The benefits of such an approach, the welfare pluralists argue, are more democracy and more efficiency or, in the view of the more economistic proponents of the 'mixed economy of welfare', greater efficiency and the more effective coordination of welfare delivery (see for example Rose, 1986; Ferlie *et al.*, 1989; Wistow *et al.*, 1992).

As advocates, the welfare pluralists are naturally more concerned with proving a case than with exploring the reasons why the private–public sector relationship in welfare takes one form rather than another. Much of their work is characterised by an acceptance of the parameters imposed by the contemporary policy debate, by a focus on outcomes (the benefits which accrue from voluntary sector involvement in service delivery), and by a neglect of the dynamic driving the policy debate in particular directions. Inevitably, therefore, the debate between welfare pluralists and traditional socialists ignores the explanatory level and is couched in terms of which approach achieves the most appropriate outcome as measured by democratic and social justice criteria. Thus Johnson, for example, judges the delivery of welfare by self-help and voluntary groups as likely to be characterised by inadequate capacity, lack of accountability and inequity of results (Johnson, 1987, 1989).

Where welfare pluralists do theorize the relationship between public and private sectors it is generally in terms of 'state failure', where non-profit organisations are seen as emerging to meet the demands of minorities not met by the state, and 'market failure', where state failure is not compensated for by market organisations (Weisbrod, 1988).

If the perspective on the private sector–NHS relationship offered by the Fabian socialists and welfare pluralists is coloured by their normative commitments, that of the quasi-market theorists is restricted by their determination to apply the principles of economic rationality to a particular set of policy developments with scant regard for the socio-political context in which those developments emerged. Taking the Conservative government's social policies from the mid-1980s onwards as their starting point, they analyse the increasing use of what they call 'quasi-market' mechanisms in the delivery of health, social care, education, and housing services. They maintain that:

> these welfare quasi-markets thus differ from conventional markets in one or more of three ways: non-profit organisations competing for public contracts, sometimes in competition with for-profit organisations; consumer purchasing power either centralised in a single purchasing agency or allocated to users in the form of vouchers rather than cash; and, in some cases, the consumers represented in the market by agents instead of operating by themselves. (Le Grand and Bartlett, 1993: 10)

Their theory is explicitly evaluative and seeks to specify 'the conditions quasi-markets will have to meet if they are to succeed, and then to make a preliminary empirical assessment of the extent to which those conditions appear to have been met in practice' (Bartlett and Le Grand, 1993: 13; see also Bartlett, 1991 and Le Grand, 1991). As this means taking a defined set of welfare policies as given and then evaluating them through the application of economic principles, it is inevitable that the boundary of the policy is the boundary of the theory. Excluded from the theory is any debate as to why the policies exist at all or why they take one form rather than another. In a not unfamiliar sequence, it is assumed without question that 'all these changes were of course the product of a Conservative government. Many of them emanated from the right-wing think-tanks that strongly influenced the ideology of that government, such as the Institute of Economic Affairs and the Adam Smith Institute' (Le Grand and Bartlett, 1993: 7). Interestingly, they do remark 'it is also worth noting' that other political parties (as well as the Conservatives) favour quasi-market policies, that other European countries are increasingly using this form of welfare service delivery, and that these changes are not confined to the public sector but are present also in private sector companies (*ibid.*: 9). However, having identified dimensions to the quasi-market issue that clearly cannot be ascribed to an omnipotent Conservative Party, they are obliged to move hurriedly on to the safety of an economic evaluation of policy implementation. Given their restricted theoretical focus, they cannot do otherwise.

Chapter 1 argued that the origins of the difficulties facing the policy-makers of the welfare state reside in the power of the values which support the policy, the historic absence of definitional limits to the social rights embodied in the concept of British citizenship, the upward spiral of expectations generated by the competition between political parties to create new categories of citizens deserving of state support, and the inability of the supply of tax revenues to keep pace with the consequent escalation in welfare demands. This theoretical perspective can be applied to the private sector and NHS relationship in order to move beyond the limitations imposed by the normative and evaluative characteristics of the approaches examined so far and to illuminate the political choices facing the state.

Logically, the most obvious strategy for a state dealing with the political problem of the demand–supply mismatch in welfare is to reduce the demands placed upon itself by persuading all citizens that they should have fewer social rights to welfare, or, at least, that they should not have additional social rights – contrary to the pattern of the past 50 years. Given the hegemony of the values of the welfare state, however, with its built-in assumptions of increasing social rights, this is at present an ideologically unacceptable approach.

A second, linked option is for the state to redirect some existing, and all additional, demand for welfare directly into the non-state or private sector. This means persuading some citizens that although their social right to welfare remains intact, as does their duty to pay for it through taxes, they may choose not to use it, or to use it only in part, and to provide for their own welfare separately and privately.

For this to happen, there has to be an ideological shift among a proportion of the citizenry to a position where the universalistic values of the welfare state are juxtaposed, but not necessarily replaced, by a belief in the importance of individual choice and self-determination and in the superior quality of private welfare. At the same time, economic incentives have to be given to the private welfare sector to increase its capacity and to citizens in order to persuade them that they should redirect their demand. However, pursuing a strategy which undermines the hegemony of welfare state values while not directly challenging that hegemony, is a difficult and dangerous tightrope for the state to walk. Because some are more able to choose private welfare than others, the charge of encouraging social inequity can readily be laid at the door of those who support the values of individual responsibility for welfare.

Third, the state can promote policies designed to blur the distinction between, on the one hand, the fulfilment of social rights through the public welfare sector and, on the other, the exercise of individual rights through the private welfare sector. The less distinct are the two sectors, the more citizens are encouraged to retreat from, or at least to reflect upon, the automatic assumption that it is the duty of the state to provide all their welfare needs; this in turn may lead to a weakening of the hegemony of welfare state values and a consequent reduction in demand for public welfare. Examples of such policies are internal markets, incentives for a mixed economy of welfare and mechanisms for attracting private finance into the public welfare arena. Also, these policies have the advantage that they emphasise the cost of welfare and the importance of the efficient use of resources in its delivery: thus, for the first time, making the relationship between the right to state welfare and its cost to the taxpayer a politically salient issue.

If the limits of state welfare have been reached but if the demand for welfare continues to expand, then the state has no choice but to pursue one or more of these three options in order to address the now pressing political problem of the demand–supply mismatch. Two of the three options involve a reassessment of the state's relationship with the private sector and, in considering the options, each political party will no doubt approach the problem differently. But no party can ignore it.

Defining the private sector and NHS relationship

At the purely descriptive level, the convention in much of the discourse about the welfare state is to divide the non-state, or private, sector into three sub-sectors: commercial, non-profit or voluntary, and informal or the family. The state, meanwhile, is generally regarded as a monolithic category. As a rhetorical aid, this view is no doubt convenient to the proponents of the perspectives discussed above but, as an analytical tool for exploring the dimensions of the political problem addressed here, is inadequate in that it fails to deal with the fluidity of the state's many boundaries. In particular, it badly underestimates the complexities of the private sector and NHS relationship.

In a rare departure from the commonly held view that the NHS is an integral part of the state, Griffith *et al.* lament the inability of their left-wing colleagues to grasp the underlying politics of health in order to be able to propel the NHS towards the socialist millenium:

> Ideological commitment – to the NHS as the jewel in Labour's crown – prevented the left from seeing the creation for what it really was: a heterogeneous range of interests and activities combined together by government intervention. Believing the health service to be a single institution – 'the NHS' – socialists forgot that it was based on public-private collaboration. (Griffith *et al.*, 1981: 106)

The NHS, they continue, has never been a monolithic, state-run system of medical care but since 1948 has relied upon a working partnership between public and private organisations. On the private side they list general practice, dentistry, opthalmic services and high-street pharmacy (self-employed professionals); pharmaceutical production and the hospital supply industries (private goods and services) (*ibid.*: 107).

The criteria used here for the inclusion of an item in the category of 'the private sector' are the common sense ones of privately employed or privately produced. It is instructive to apply these simple criteria to the 1995 *Health and Personal Social Services Statistics for England* to gain a general idea of the private sector's presence within current NHS expenditure (see Table 8.1).

The NHS has always been made up of a mix of private and public provision and the proportions have remained stable over the past 50 years as the core of state-employed staff in hospitals has continued to balance the other, private, categories of provision. Once the myth of the NHS as a monolithic state institution is replaced by the reality of a substantial private sector presence *within* the NHS, debate becomes more meaningful, a reasonably level playing field is established, and the carefully nurtured illusions of public sector purity less of an analytical hindrance.

Table 8.1 Expenditure on the NHS 1994 – private and public sector provision

	£ million	%
Private Sector	**16630**	**53**
General Practitioner	2507	
Pharmaceutical	3656	
General Dental	1222	
General Opthalmic	192	
Supplies equipment, services	8182	
Capital projects	618	
Agency staff	253	
Public Sector	**14645**	**47**
NHS staff salaries and wages	13660	
Other (e.g. administration)	985	
Total	**31275**	**100**

Source: Health and Personal Social Services (1995: section VII, Tables 7.1, 7.4 and 7.9).

Drawing on the concepts of demand and supply used to delineate the political problem summarised in Chapter 1 (Figure 1.3), the financial demand for health care can be divided into public and private categories and set against the public and private provision of health care thus creating a four cell typology (Figure 8.1).

	Financial Demand	
	Private	*Public*
Provision		
Private	1	2
Public	3	4

Figure 8.1 Typology of the private and public sector relationship

The categories are:

1. Private insurance companies or individuals purchasing their health care from private providers.
2. Publicly funded agencies (HAs, GP Fundholders, or NHS Trusts) contracting services from the private sector: for example, clinical provision (for example waiting list initiatives), pharmaceutical supplies, laundry and catering. This category includes the policies of 'contracting out' and 'competitive tendering'.
3. Private insurance and other companies and individuals purchasing their health care and other services from publicly owned providers (Trusts): for example, paybeds and 'income generation schemes'.
4. Publicly funded agencies contracting health care from publicly owned organisations (Trusts). This includes inter-Trust trading.

The application of the typology to selected markets, or client groups, in health care demonstrates both the extent and the variety of the mixed economy of health care that already exists (Table 8.2.).

Whilst some markets are dominated by the single category of public finance and public supply (elective surgery, acute psychiatric, maternity), in others there is a distribution across two categories of the mixed economy (psychiatric rehabilitation, long-term mentally ill and mentally handicapped), three categories (abortions) and four categories (elderly residential long-term care).

For the state, the development of a private–public mix in welfare raises further important issues regarding the political management of its delivery. If it is to move to a position where it can use its adjustment of the private–public mix of welfare as a political means for dealing with the problem of the excess demand for welfare over the available supply, then clearly it requires the financial and legal leverage to achieve this end as well as the accountability mechanisms to ensure that the public's taxes are used appropriately in terms of both allocative process and policy outcomes. Yet too much bureaucratic control will stifle the endeavour in its infancy and inhibit private sector involvement. How can the state resolve this dilemma?

Table 8.2 The mixed economy of health care in selected markets

MARKET	*Year to which relates*	*Data base*	*Category 1 Private finance, private supply %*	*Category 2 Public finance, private supply %*	*Category 3 Private finance, public supply %*	*Category 4 Public finance, public supply %*
Elective surgery	1992/93	Cases	11.9	0.2	1.5	86.4
Elderly residential long-term care	1995	Cash	37	32.5	2.5	28
Acute psychiatric	1995	Beds	5	2	small	93
Psychiatric rehabilitation, long-term mentally ill	1995	Beds	small	61	small	39
Long-term mentally handicapped	1995	Beds	small	55	small	45
Maternity	1994	Births	1	small	small	99
Abortions	1995	Cases	36	16	small	48

Source: Laing and Buisson, 1996: Table 1.3, A62.

Managing the private sector and NHS relationship

While the imperative to manage the private–public welfare mix is now an inescapable fact of political life, it must also be recognised that other, objective, characteristics of contemporary public administration render a continuing review of that mix a necessary part of modern government. In discussing the accountability dimensions of the move from what she terms the 'Provider State' to the 'Regulatory State', Day observes:

> the developments of the 1980s cannot sensibly be seen as the product merely of Thatcherite market ideology: if we ignore the long-term trends towards the' breakdown of the public-private distinction', as a way of solving the problems of complexity in modern government, we miss much of the significance of what happened. (Day, 1992: 6)

The large and diverse responsibilities of modern government require delivery systems more flexible than the old-style, hierarchical model of public administration is able to provide. Out of this need grew the Financial Management Initiative and the Next Steps Initiative – both of which sought to transform the way in which Whitehall worked, to break down the rigidities inherent in traditional bureaucracies and to utilise private sector skills and capacities where appropriate (Greer, 1994). Such developments parallel others which have already occurred in the private sector. As early as the 1950s and 1960s, private firms discovered the benefits of 'contracting out' some of their functions in order to take advantage of the flexibility offered by the increasing specialisation of labour and more competitive pricing in the rapidly growing service industries (Ascher, 1987: 19).

Although it can be argued that it was only a question of time before these apparent opportunities for injecting greater efficiency into the organisation of state services produced some kind of effect, such changes will always have to pass through the filters of party ideology, political self-interest and bureaucratic resistance. In terms of its political value, therefore, 'administrative efficiency' still has a relative, not an absolute, status. But with the increasing salience of the mismatch between citizen expectations of welfare and the state sponsored supply, this relative status has improved as the political utility of new forms of welfare delivery systems has become steadily more apparent. Policies dealing with competitive tendering, contracting out, 'harnessing the private sector' and so on, have gradually acquired respectability as their administrative and political advantage have been seen to coincide.

It has been an uneven process. In central government, the contracting out of services has never received the attention or the obloquy heaped on the policy at the local level. In 1979, after two decades of largely Labour government, 85 per cent of all cleaning in central departments of state was carried out by private contractors as the result of a policy originally initiated in 1968 (*ibid.*: 25 and 43). In contrast to this, Ascher has charted the arduous journey of the Conservatives' policy on the contracting out of ancillary services in the Health Service. The original 1980 circular *Revised guidance on contractual arrangements and cooperative schemes* was brusquely rebuffed by Health Authorities and subsequent circulars met with, at best, grudging acceptance and, at worst, circuitous delaying manoeuvres (*ibid.*). Likewise, the income generation initiative, begun by the

1988 Health and Medicines Act which allowed NHS hospitals to sell their clinical support services to the private sector and keep any profit, was by 1991–92 still only producing an estimated £25 million per year of extra income and performance was what the National Audit Office termed 'patchy' (National Audit Office, 1993: 6).

Selling clinical services themselves, in the form of NHS paybeds, to the private sector has traditionally been the most emotive of the private–public sector issues and the one least amenable to consensus politics. The 1975–79 Labour government set up the Health Service Board to phase out paybeds and the Conservative government's 1980 Health Services Act duly abolished the Board. At the same time, the Conservatives used the regulatory powers of the state to encourage change in the private–public mix of welfare by promoting the growth of the private health care sector. Tax incentives were provided for the purchase of private health insurance, consultants' contracts were altered in order to facilitate their private practice, and the planning restrictions on private hospital developments were relaxed (Mohan and Woods, 1985; Rayner, 1986). A moderate expansion of private provision ensued in the decade following the 1979 election, with the number of private hospitals increasing by 39 per cent and private beds by 58 per cent (Calnan *et al.*, 1993: 4). On the demand side, the proportion of the population with private health insurance increased from 5 to 13 per cent in the same period (*ibid.*: 2–3).

By the late 1980s, the limits of the two strands of Conservative policy designed to change the balance of the welfare mix in health had clearly been reached. In the NHS, bureaucratic inertia had successfully taken the steam out of the contracting out policy so that whereas, in 1984, 74 per cent of contracts for ancillary services were awarded to private companies, by 1990, 77 per cent went to in-house bids (McGregor, 1990). Income generation was thus far a non-event and in the period 1981–89 paybeds had only barely increased from 2700 to 3000 (bearing in mind that in 1971 there had been 4400 paybeds) (Central Statistical Office, 1993: 108). Meanwhile in the private health care sector there was an over-supply of beds coupled with low occupancy rates (Calnan *et al.*, 1993: 3), and the proportion of the population privately insured had peaked at its 1989–90 figure of 13 per cent and was now, if not in decline, certainly very flat (Central Statistical Office, 1994: 105). If the state's management of the welfare mix was to have any substantial impact in the future, clearly something completely different had to be tried.

While it is unlikely that the 1989 NHS Review was a conscious and rational response to the perceived inadequacies of the private–public sector policies on health pursued up to this point, wittingly or otherwise, it created a fresh dynamic for change which has yet to run its course. The 1990 NHS and Community Care Act established the framework for a market in health care, funded and managed by the state. Within this market, purchasing agencies (Health Authorities and GP Fundholders), acting on behalf of citizens, contracted health care from provider organisations (NHS Trusts and others). Although the policy was initially described as establishing a market *internal* to the NHS, later government statements made it plain that it very much encouraged trading across NHS and private sector boundaries. Returning now to Figure 8.1, we can see that this meant potentially expanded activity in categories 2 and 3 and potentially reduced activity in categories 1 and 4. What impact on the mixed economy of health care has the policy actually had?

In terms of category 2 (public finance and private supply), disappointingly little from the private sector's perspective. The expectation that private hospitals could make inroads into the provision of clinical services for the NHS has not materialised. NHS purchasers have not established what the private sector regards as an appropriate 'contract culture' and have largely remained faithful to their NHS providers (Laing and Buisson, 1996: A80). (GP fundholder income, of which the private hospitals had high hopes, in 1995 accounted for perhaps 2 per cent of independent hospitals' and clinics' £1.3 billion turnover (*ibid.*).) There is the strong suspicion among private sector operators that a level playing field does not exist and that:

> the role of the private sector in NHS service delivery will only grow significantly to the extent that NHS purchasers become willing to consider contracting out lumps of service where cost comparisons between independent and NHS provision incorporate capital investment and overheads. (*ibid.*)

In the meantime, many private acute service providers are reluctant to expend management time in what they anticipate will be abortive discussions with the NHS.

They also have to contend with the impact of the reforms on category 3 (private finance and public supply). The NHS and Community Care Act was even-handed in its liberating treatment of private and public providers of health care. For the private sector it removed the requirement that it should seek permission for the building of any hospital with more than 120 beds. For the public sector it removed the final curbs on pay beds: in future no authorisation was required from Health Authorities or the Secretary of State for those hospitals wishing to establish pay beds to do so. NHS Trusts have taken advantage of this to develop or improve their dedicated pay bed units which, although small in number, have made inroads into the private acute health care market. NHS private patient income rose from £83 million in 1988 to £230 million in 1995 and its share of the private acute health care market from 11.2 per cent to 15.1 per cent over the same period (*ibid.*, Table 2.7, A84). Some private insurers, notably Norwich Union, have contracts with NHS Trusts to guarantee their customers treatment in NHS private beds (*Health Service Journal*, 1994a).

Although the NHS's share of the private acute hospital market has increased, a different picture emerges when we look at the relative sizes of the private and public sectors in terms of combined hospital and nursing home supply. Expressed as a percentage of total private and NHS supply, the private sector's share of this market has increased from 9.9 per cent in 1986 to 19.8 per cent in 1995 (Laing and Buisson, 1996: Table 1.1, A60). The increase is due to the rapid expansion of private nursing home provision prompted by the discovery of open-ended social security support for the elderly and the corresponding decrease in NHS provision. Once that loophole was closed with the implemention of the NHS and Community Care Act in 1992, little further increase has occurred. So there has been a trade-off between the NHS's improved acute hospital market share and the private sector's improved nursing home market share with the balance of the overall advantage going to the private sector.

As the two-way flows across the boundaries of the private sector and NHS increase, and equally importantly are seen to increase, so the state's imperative to divert and to limit the demands of the citizenry upon the state's finite welfare resources becomes more of a realisable political option. But for the process to arrive at a successful conclusion, sophisticated political management is required. The key question is one of the balance of control: how can the requirements of public accountability be achieved while permitting the freedoms necessary for any market mechanism to work across the boundaries of the private–public sector relationship?

The means which the state has at its disposal for the political management of health care delivery within the NHS include the formal accountability mechanisms of the Public Accounts Committee and the Audit Commission (focusing in particular on issues of probity), the general management and corporate contract system of the NHS, and the Secretary of State's direct access to Health Authority and Trust chairs. Much grist has also been added to the accountability mill by the impact of the Nolan Committee on standards in public life and the growing emphasis within the Health Service on the appropriate procedures of corporate governance. What is only just now emerging as an issue, however, is how and to what extent the state regulates not only what happens *within* the Health Service but also *between* the NHS and the private sector and, if necessary, *within* the private sector itself.

Historically, the accountability of the private sector for the services it provides to the NHS has been achieved through a commercial contract. Whether this will continue to be an appropriate control device if the private sector's provider share of NHS and other public expenditure on health care continues to increase must be regarded as unlikely, because the state will still require short-term adjustments in NHS activity (for example on waiting lists) for party political purposes, as well as guarantees that public money is being used efficiently and effectively. Furthermore, should the private insurance market expand significantly from its present static base of 13 per cent of the population, there will come a point where the state is obliged to take rather more of an interest than it does at present in the regulation of the processes and outcomes of this market. Private pensions and their potential contribution to the costs of elderly care are areas where this issue is beginning to surface: for example in the consultation document *A new partnership for care in old age* (Chancellor of the Exchequer *et al.*, 1996).

More likely, therefore, is the creation of auditing procedures specifically designed to deal with a mixed economy of health care, coupled with powers to take corrective action where required. In other policy areas such as housing this has already led to the development of new types of bureaucratic control using semi-independent monitoring agencies (Day, 1992: 15). In this context it is instructive to explore in some detail the accountability issues which have arisen in the course of the implementation of the Private Finance Initiative (PFI) in the NHS.

The Private Finance Initiative

The Private Finance Initiative was launched in 1992 across all government departments with the objective of increasing the relatively minor commitment of private capital to public schemes. There are three types of PFI scheme:

1. The costs of the project are funded entirely by private money and recovered by means of direct charges to the end user.
2. The private sector funds the project and recoups its costs by selling the services the facility provides mainly or entirely to the public sector.
3. The capital cost is divided between public and private funds with overall responsibility for the project resting with the private sector (Treasury Committee of the House of Commons, 1996: viii).

In (1) and (2) the overall effect is to shift capital expenditure into current expenditure via payments for services. The political advantage of this is that because the public sector contracts to buy services not assets, the capital expenditure thus achieved does not form part of the Public Sector Borrowing Requirement (PSBR) – hence allowing the state greater short-term spending flexibility. In the long term the effect of the policy is that the costs of investment are passed to future years (and future taxpayers) but this implication has not so far acted to diminish the immediate attractions of the policy to politicians of all parties. Public sector capital expenditure is projected to fall by £2.5 billion between 1995–96 and 1998–99 and as a proportion of Gross Domestic Product (GDP) from 1.75 per cent in 1995–96 to 0.75 per cent in 2000–01 (*ibid.*: ix). Effectively, PFI schemes are to replace orthodox public capital spending.

The application of the Private Finance Initiative to the Health Service has raised new accountability issues not normally encountered in its trading relationships with the private sector. As PFI has unfolded, it has become clear that the big PFI ventures are not so much building contracts as very large, long-term service contracts involving a multiplicity of participants organised in consortia which generate quite novel regulatory problems for the state. PFI is about considerably more than simply 'private finance'. It is about the detailed web of commercial relationships which must exist in order to render the use of that finance viable for both private and public partners. Where exactly does the public interest sit within this maze of relationships and how should the state seek to protect it? Second, and more problematically, to what extent is it in the public interest for the state to cultivate and sustain a private sector capable of providing the NHS with the capital infrastructure it has always lacked?

The continuing search for an answer to these questions is clearly evident in the Financial Directive Letters (FDLs) issued by the National Health Service Executive (NHSE), with a strong input from the PFI section of the Treasury, offering guidance to Trusts interested in pursuing the private finance option (Salter and Douglas, 1994). Embedded within these documents is a political subtext of risk management and hints of the struggle between those in the Conservative party who wished to give greater rein to the private sector's involvement in the NHS (see Willetts, 1993), and others such as Treasury officials who were, and are, concerned that the process should be closely regulated.

The FDL issued in January 1993 set out the Treasury's interim guidance and confirmed that the 'private sector is to be actively encouraged to take the lead in joint ventures with the public sector.... The NHS will still have to demonstrate value for money... but where the private sector is in the lead, it will no longer be necessary to consider a theoretical alternative funded wholly by the NHS'. Value for money and the sharing of risk were emphasised as being key criteria (NHSE, 1993d). This was followed by an FDL on approval procedures which gave the Finance and Corporate Information Directorate of the NHSE a discretionary power which might or might not facilitate, probably depending on the Treasury view, the emergence of schemes into the light of day (NHSE, 1993e). Committee drafting was evident. On the one hand, the FDL cautiously observed that 'the use of private finance needs to be controlled because it can, in some cases, be more expensive than using public capital'. And, on the other, it pronounced that the 'use of private sector entrepreneurial skills and management disciplines can spur innovation, effectiveness, efficiency and better managed risks' (*ibid.*). The third FDL, which dealt specifically with leasing arrangements with the private sector, then developed the risk argument further. Its premise was that there is little attraction to the government in leasing if it simply represents deferred purchase and that it will usually be cheaper to finance the purchase directly. For leasing to be value for money, therefore, it must be shown that there is a net transfer of risk to the private sector combined with improved asset management which together exceed the additional cost of leasing (NHSE, 1993f).

As with most government guidance on NHS links with the private sector, the preoccupation in these early FDLs was how best to ensure that public money and the public interest are adequately protected through the use of appropriate systems of accountability. Little attention was paid to the other side of the coin: the obstacles that lie in the path of private sector commitment to such agreements and how these might be removed. Interestingly, in its consultative document *Financing Infrastructure Investment: Promoting a Partnership Between Public and Private Finance* the Labour Party took the Conservative government to task for not being more pro-active in removing these obstacles. In particular, it was critical of the Conservative government's failure to remove a number of uncertainties faced by the private sector. First, the open tendering procedure which a private company is obliged to endure acts as a disincentive and 'often raises serious issues of intellectual property rights and design expenditure' (Labour Party, 1994: 10). Second, there is little guidance on how the majority of risk is to be transferred to the private company and forcing the transfer of too much risk may cause the private sector to withdraw or may simply push up costs (*ibid.*).

In the case of prospective agreements between the private sector and NHS Trusts, a third ambiguity was present in the uncertainties surrounding the legal status and powers of Trusts and hence their reliability for business purposes (Long and Salter, 1994). In response to private sector enquiries about this issue, the NHSE published a fourth FDL which sought to clarify the position for those private companies interested in joint ventures with Trusts but which succeeded only in muddying the waters still further (NHSE, 1993f). While private companies may have been reassured by the statement that 'the aim is to ensure that a Trust does not fail financially' and that the NHSE would intervene if there was a danger of a Trust getting into severe financial difficulties, they would certainly have been alarmed by the further information that the Secretary of State need not honour all of the contractual liabilities of a Trust which is dissolved (and 'this can happen without consultation') but would exercise his/her 'discretion over what property, rights and liabilities are recognised' (*ibid.*). While this clause reduced the risk to the public sector organisation of an agreement with the private sector, it also increased the risk to the private company and reflected the dominant drift at this time in the state's handling of the private–public relationship. In due course the NHS (Residual Liabilities) Act 1996 was introduced to reassure the private sector that the government would honour the liabilities of a Trust which is dissolved, but initially the question of responsibilities to the private sector did not form part of the bureaucratic agenda.

Observers pointed out that the issue the state had not addressed was what legal, tax and other incentives could be put into place in order to encourage private sector support for NHS capital projects and control the risk to which the private partners are exposed (*Health Service Journal*, 1994b). Pressure for the state to do so mounted as the momentum behind its withdrawal from the public funding of capital projects became evident and the corresponding dependence upon private money became inevitable. In 1994 *The Capital Investment Manual* was issued by the NHSE providing detailed guidance on the procedures governing NHS capital projects (NHSE, 1994h). To it had been added at a late stage the rule that every such business case should show that serious consideration had been given to the PFI option: PFI was now in the procedural mainstream and effectively blocked the Trusts' route to Treasury money. Further guidance on testing the PFI option was issued the following year in which Trusts were pointed in the direction of a specific model of their relationship with a private partner:

> An option that many projects will need to explore is one in which the private sector would undertake the design, building, financing and operation of the non-clinical services [or 'DBFO' schemes]. An NHS Trust's role in such a scheme could include a commitment to using the building for the provision of health care services for NHS patients for an agreed period. The Trust would therefore manage and provide all the health care services, while the private partner could provide the fully serviced building. (NHSE, 1995e: 5)

Clearly the intention was to promote large, whole hospital projects, which up to this point had been conspicuous by their absence, rather than the small facilities projects such as waste incinerators which had so far constituted the staple diet of PFI. In the same year, information management and technology procurement was also swept into the PFI net (NHSE, 1995f).

The imperative that the rules governing the private–public relationship in PFI should be made to work, and work efficiently, was reinforced by the November 1995 budget. A pronounced whiff of burning bridges surrounded the Chancellor's announcement that there was to be a 16.9 per cent cut in the financing of the hospital building programme and that the shortfall was to be made up by PFI (Gulland, 1996: 18). Given the experience up to this point, if this was indeed to happen the flexibility of the PFI bureaucracy would have to be considerably enhanced. By June 1996 the government was claiming that 'there are now 57 approved PFI projects with a capital value of more than £500 million, including four major district hospitals' (DoH, 1996c). The reality, however, was that at that time none of the larger 'approved' schemes had been finalised because of their sheer complexity and the delays inherent in negotiating a way through the labyrinthe of PFI procedures. Only one information technology project worked its way through PFI in 1995. The rest were sent back to square one (*Health Service Journal*, 1996).

The Private Finance Initiative has the potential to rearrange the private–public mix in health care into a qualitatively new form and balance. In the long term, the implication of the design, build, finance and operate (DBFO) approach is that although core clinical services will be given the status of protected territory all other services involved in the delivery of health care may be owned and/or managed by the private sector. As yet the state has only just begun to untangle the implications of such arrangements for its political management of the NHS and is groping for the appropriate balance between accountability, governance and control, on the one hand, and freedom, flexibility and invention, on the other. Furthermore, it does not speak with a single voice. In its scrutiny of PFI the Treasury Committee of the House of Commons did not agree with the government's view that the details of PFI contracts should not be publicly available:

> We do not think that the House would or should sacrifice its rights to see any details of Government spending it sees fit. We stress that the Government's duty to account for its spending to the House is not conditional upon the House's willingness not to disclose such information; if the House refused to give such assurances, it would be improper for the Government to withold details it regarded as commercially confidential, and unlikely that the House would accept that, in such cases, the accounting officer's satisfaction that value for money had been achieved was sufficient. (Treasury Committee of the House of Commons, 1996: xxi)

In many ways the debate has only just begun.

Conclusions

In confronting the problem of the mismatch between the demand for state welfare generated by the ever-growing array of social rights embodied in the concept of British citizenship and the finite supply of public finance from its taxpayers, the state has to deal with a complex set of political issues. Technically, its options are, first, to limit or reduce demand by restrictions on social rights; second, to divert demand by inducing citizens to finance their welfare privately; or, third, to attempt to do both by a blurring of the boundaries between the private and public sectors of welfare. Whichever option, or combination of options, is selected will require a redefinition of the welfare state not only as a policy but, more importantly, as a central component of British political culture.

The dominance of traditional welfare state values, of the political expectations which are embedded within them and of the electoral calculations they promote, render ideological change a necessary companion of any realistic policy initiatives. Social policy observers have shown themselves to be as susceptible as any to the analytical blinkers imposed by this hegemony and, consequently, as impervious to the critical political problem that that same hegemony has created. In their anxiety to maintain that hegemony and in their haste to sustain the illusion of a public health care system unsullied by private provision, they have failed to analyse, or perhaps to realise, the extent to which there has always been a mixed economy of state-financed health care. Achieving an unconscious symmetry, their negative view of the private sector is a mirror image of the unreflective enthusiasm for the private domain which characterises the attitude of the New Right.

Historically, the NHS has always been an amalgam of private and public provision and trading across the private and public sector boundaries an accepted and continuing feature of the British health care system. Until the 1980s, the myth of a wholly public NHS was not challenged and therefore there was no ideological need to review the way in which the state covertly managed, or did not manage, the private sector and NHS relationship. But as the tension between the demand for health care and the available supply has grown, and with it the political need for a reappraisal of the private–public relationship, so the state has been obliged to place the functions of finance, provision and regulation on the explicit political agenda. To an extent the policies on contracting out and competitive tendering simply delayed the state's hand in this matter because they were seen as in some sense exceptional.

Each of the three options available to the state requires that the hegemony of traditional values is challenged. The last two options (demand diversion and boundary obfuscation) also dictate that the state reflects not only on its preferred mix of private and public finance, and private and public provision, for the delivery of health care but also on the appropriate means of the state management of this mix. For no matter how radical are the solutions offered, the state will still retain responsibility for ensuring that the system as a whole works and that its publicly financed component is adequately monitored.

Visible changes in the traditional balance of the mixed economy of health care serve to illuminate the fact that the private–public boundaries exist, are shifting and are deserving of monitoring and regulation. However, the effect of the 1991 reforms on that mix was scarcely dramatic. Category 2 of the typology of the private–public relationship (public finance, private supply) expanded but little and category 3 (private finance, public supply) showed the NHS Trusts' pay beds making some inroads into the private insurance market. Ironically, the most vibrant area of private sector supply, nursing homes, found its growth capped by the 1990 Act's removal of the social security loophole on which it had relied since the early 1980s. Instead, the most significant force for change in the state's political management of the private–public relationship has been the Private Finance Initiative.

PFI represents a potential sea-change in the way in which the state funds the capital infrastructure of the welfare state in general and the NHS in particular. Its importance lies not so much in the use of private finance itself as in the framework of unique legal and commercial relationships on which the use of that finance is contingent. The framework not only has to guarantee the private sector partners that they have a viable business proposition sustainable over a period of, frequently, several decades but also has to reassure the NHS partners that risk is transferred, value for money obtained and the requirements of public accountability achieved. Such a complex and enduring framework is unprecedented in the history of the private sector and Health Service relationship and is taking time to evolve into a workable bureaucratic form which can readily be applied to different PFI projects. Once established for a given project, however, it will be impossible to unravel without either a high political cost as the service is withdrawn or a substantial input of fresh public capital – neither of which are feasible courses of action in the current and foreseeable political climate.

Of its very nature, PFI achieves the objective of the state's third option of blurring the boundary between the private and public health sectors. The interdependence of the private and public partners is legally binding, money flows both ways and services are traded. Equally, the very fluidity of PFI highlights the inappropriateness of the traditional state mechanisms for monitoring and managing the mixed economy of health care. It is to the development of more sophisticated and flexible systems of accountability that the state is obliged to look in its handling of the private–public relationship.

9

Conclusions

Introduction

The politics of change in the Health Service are a product of enduring aspects of British citizenship and political culture. It is this context which presents the polity with the fundamental political problem of welfare, circumscribes any policy response to that problem by the state and determines the nature of subsequent policy interaction with the NHS power structures.

Previous chapters have sought to illuminate the impact of this process on the power relations of the NHS, as it is the balance of forces between these interests, alliances and antagonisms which constitute the true measure of political change. In this concluding chapter, a reckoning is made of where the equilibrium now rests between the principal players of politicians, managers, bureaucrats and doctors in the various theatres of Health Service engagement.

It is preceded by a restatement of the guiding thesis of this book, the lesson of which is that the politicisation of the NHS is here to stay. The die is cast, and regardless of the party in government the Health Service will continue to be a high profile political issue, generating policies which will reverberate against its power structures.

The problem of citizenship

Enoch Powell observed that 'no social benefit once conferred can ever be withdrawn'. Behind this statement lie a set of assumptions about the nature of British citizenship which combine to produce the political problem facing the welfare state in general and the NHS in particular. The welfare state is the chosen vehicle for the delivery of the social rights embodied in British citizenship. Whereas civil and political rights are generally formulated in a negative way in terms of freedom 'from' (mostly from state intervention), social rights are formulated in a positive way requiring an interventionist state to achieve them. Furthermore, they are given an absolute status and their fulfilment is not seen as conditional upon the ability of the state, primarily its economic ability, to provide them. Rather the state is seen as having the absolute duty to deliver the welfare component of citizenship, regardless of the costs.

The National Health Service was founded to provide British citizens with their health care rights. From its inception, these rights were regarded as unfettered by any restrictive definition of health or any notion of the limits to the state's responsibilities. As a result, the concept of 'the healthy citizen' with their full quota of health rights is an elastic concept which can be readily adapted to include a range of physical, psychological, psychiatric, and social characteristics in order to suit the needs of particular interest groups. At the same time, the symbiotic relationship between citizen rights and state duties was reinforced by the tax-financed, integrated state provision model adopted by the NHS. In contrast to this 'Beveridge' model of health care delivery, many European countries introduced the social insurance 'Bismarck' model, where the insurance funds may be to a considerable extent independent of government (Taylor-Gooby, 1996). In political terms, the significance of the continuum between the Beveridge and Bismarck models is the distance it represents between citizen rights and state duties. The closer a health care delivery system is to the Beveridge model, the tighter the rights–duties nexus and the less freedom of manoeuvre there is available to the state. The more a state takes responsibility for the functions of finance, provision and regulation the greater its political exposure to the legitimate demands of its citizens. To put it another way, if there were no health care rights the health of the nation would not be a political problem.

The translation of health care rights into demands upon the political system is influenced by the interaction between the ideology of the welfare state and the characteristics of party politics in an electoral democracy. Welfare state values constitute an hegemony within which political parties must operate if they are to achieve electoral success. Inherent in these values is the assumption that welfare rights can be increased, or at least maintained, but certainly not diminished. Any slackening of the demand registered by these rights is therefore opposed by the hegemony. Instead, the incentive is for parties to compete to create new rights and hence new demands upon the polity. In the case of the Health Service, this has meant, for example, the invention of the Patient's Charter with its panoply of national monitoring arrangements, the evolution of the Health of the Nation programme into a target-setting exercise, the issuing by the DoH of numerous priority 'wish lists' (Health Committee of the House of Commons, 1995: xvii) and the introduction of invigorated complaints procedures to report unfulfilled rights.

None of this would constitute a political problem for the state if its resources were sufficient to meet the demand thus generated. The growth in the supply of tax revenues, however, has never kept pace with the growth in the demands on the welfare state and with taxation now at its electorally acceptable upper limit the salience of the demand–supply mismatch is inescapable. The government is caught in a cleft stick of political costs: it can either increase taxation and lose votes or fail to meet the demand for welfare and lose votes.

The hegemony of welfare renders it difficult, if not illegitimate, for the state to make choices between competing claims for health care resources on behalf of the public interest – in other words, to engage in what the public choice theorists would regard as the normal business of government (see for example Ranson and Stewart, 1989). In the NHS this difficulty was traditionally handled by the medical profession through the exercise of covert rationing legitimised by clinical judgement and it was the performance of the key function of managing the demand–supply mismatch which formed, and forms, the basis of medical power. But in the absence of a price or other mechanism for giving expressed demand an individual cost and regulating the demand–supply relationship, the demand for state health care consistently outstripped the available supply despite the covert rationing by doctors. Evidence of the mismatch were waiting lists, the diversion of unmet demand to the private sector and the consequent expansion of the private insurance market in the 1980s, and the rising tide of formal complaints about the Health Service from the early eighties onwards (Klein, 1995: 306–8).

In response to the increasingly visible political problem at the heart of the Health Service, the Conservative government established the 1989 Review of the NHS. Disregarding its original brief, the Review decided that the demand side of the equation (the consideration of alternative forms of funding state health care) was too difficult and concentrated exclusively on the supply side. *Working for Patients* therefore dealt with organisational changes designed to alleviate the pressures on the service through improved operational efficiency which subsequent guidance revealed was to be achieved through a quasi-market mechanism. What effect did these changes have on the distribution of power in the NHS?

The balance of power

Before the 1989 Review, policy-making on the NHS was dominated by the long-standing alliance between the central Department and the medical profession. Born out of the concordat between the state and the profession on which the foundation of the NHS was contingent, the alliance was designed to ensure that the major producer interest of the Health Service was appropriately consulted and incorporated in any significant policy decision (Ham, 1985: 97–9). Although individual doctors may have felt threatened by the general management reforms that were introduced after the 1983 Griffiths Report was published, the profession's elites remained secure in their unique access to the apparatus of state power.

The Review changed all that. Consultation between it and the medical profession was non-existent. From a privileged position at the centre of health policy affairs, doctors' organisations found themselves suddenly thrust to the pluralistic margins with all the other lobby groups. On top of the indignity of such treatment, the profession was then presented with a White Paper which clearly intended that in the search for operational efficiency doctors should be subject to similar requirements of management accountability as other NHS staff (DoH, 1989a). Commissioning agencies (primarily District Health Authorities [DHAs]) were to identify the needs of their local populations and contract the services to meet those needs from competing self-governing hospital Trusts endowed with a new range of management and financial freedoms. The tradition of 'producer capture' of the Health Service by the medical profession was to be replaced by a needs-driven approach to health care which would make the service more responsive to patients. So far as the key actors in the new scenario were concerned, *Working for Patients* was clear that its proposals were building on the general management structures already established (*ibid.*: 11). These would be used 'to ensure that consultants are properly accountable for the consequences of [their] decisions', that medical audit was appropriately developed, and that the consultant's job contract and distinction awards (once reformed) were suitably managed (*ibid.*: Ch. 5). In terms of formal policy intent, NHS managers were in pole position.

It was expected that operational managers would drive the organisational reforms and, *ipso facto*, achieve the redistribution of power on which the stated aims of the policy of the 'internal market', as it became known, depended. Despite the commercial rhetoric which accompanied the reforms, however, there was never any doubt that the characteristics which distinguish management of organisations in the public domain from those in the private sector would play a vital part in the post-1991 NHS. As Ranson and Stewart have observed, the tendency of organisational models to define many activities of public bodies (protest, politics, public accountability, citizenship, party conflict, elections, public debate, inter-authority cooperation, and civil rights) as either without the concerns of management or as interferences ('efficiency has to be sacrificed for democracy', 'the constraints of public accountability', 'the costs of democracy') fails to understand the nature of public management (Ranson and Stewart, 1989: 5). They continue:

> those dimensions which are conceptualised as constraints upon effective organisational working are in fact qualities of value or constitutive conditions within public organisations. A concept of organisation that encompasses citizens differs from an organisation that knows only customers. Thus a concept of management is needed which encompasses the recognition of political difference and conflict as constitutive of a public organisation rather than an obstacle to it (*ibid.*: 5–6).

In the first flush of enthusiasm which accompanied the introduction of the internal market, many NHS managers confused rhetoric with reality and were persuaded that they could indeed act with the independence accorded to managers of private organisations. Such a view sadly overestimated the ability of formal policy to alter the web of power relations within the Health Service, founded as they are on the fundamental requirement to control and regulate citizens' expectations. In particular it underestimated the need of ministers to retain firm levers of control at all levels.

As the national focal point for the political expression of those expectations, consecutive Secretaries of State for Health found it impossible to diminish their level of responsibility for the health care service simply by changing the manner in which it was delivered.

Greater devolution of operational control to the local level did not, in the eyes of the public, mean that accountability for the fulfilment of their health care rights was transferred as well. The NHS is, by definition, a national not a local service with a centralised system of management accountability leading directly to the Secretary of State. In the absence of a local democratic tier to hive off local grievances, political pressure on the Health Service from its citizens must be channelled to the national level. Such pressure is frequently harnessed and magnified by local MPs who, given the electoral sensitivity of the NHS, have never been slow to lobby the Minister on behalf of their constituents.

In order to respond effectively to the many and varied pressures thus generated, Department of Health (DoH) ministers must retain the capacity for both strategic and tactical intervention in the Health Service. For this they need a bureaucracy. Thus it was the case that at the same time as operational responsibilities were being devolved to Trust managers, the lines of accountability between Health Authorities, regions and the National Health Service Executive (NHSE) remained very much intact, reinforced by the Secretary of State's personal line of influence through regional, Health Authority and Trust chairs.

The continuing need for controls and the bureaucrats to operate them has been augmented by ministers' masochistic tendency to encourage fresh demands to be placed on the NHS (and thus themselves); by fears that market mechanisms may undermine public accountability; and by certain objective characteristics of the Health Service as a whole.

Under the heady influence of the welfare state hegemony, politicians compete to give citizens more social rights. In the case of the NHS, this urge has found particularly effective expression in the Patients' Charter. Once in place, the Charter required a bureaucracy, largely administered by the Health Authorities, to sustain its impetus and monitor its achievements as a vehicle for fulfilling, as well as arousing, citizen expectations. A small industry developed around this demand-creation function and through the visibility of the issues it generated (for example via league tables of hospitals' performance) ensured that bureaucratic controls were *in situ* to persuade underperforming Trusts to adjust their activities in order to attain the desired targets.

Second, the need to maintain financial probity through appropriate bureaucratic mechanisms did not diminish simply because of a policy shift in health care delivery. Indeed, the House of Commons Public Accounts Committee has made it abundantly clear that the relationship between public money and quasi-market funding mechanisms has to be closely monitored precisely because it departs from traditional modes of expenditure, and that this is particularly the case where the private sector is involved. Governance, as it has become known, is now a permanent feature of the NHS's political agenda. If it were needed, further fuel to the issue has been added by the Nolan Committee and its concern that public service values should not be undermined by new forms of public service delivery. Ensuring that these values remain intact of course requires, as always, more guidance and more monitoring. In the case of dealings with the private sector, the effect of this climate of risk avoidance is the proliferation of bureaucratic protocols. Only a cursory glance is required at the procedures which have mushroomed around the Private Finance Initiative to be reassured that bureaucracy is alive and well in the Health Service.

Probity is one bureaucratic function that has had to be retained, planning is another. Even in the early days of the 1991 reforms it was accepted that some 'management of the market' was required but it was assumed that this could be kept to a minimum. What has steadily become apparent, however, is that there are certain objective characteristics of the NHS which demand a planning input and without which unacceptably high political costs will be incurred in terms of disruptions to existing service provision. Taking medical manpower as an example, the combined impact of the New Deal for junior doctors and the Calman reforms of postgraduate medical education has created an objective need for cross-Trust collaboration in the management of change in the delivery of the new training. More intensive training requires a reorientation, if not a relocation, of service provision, supported by appropriate commissioning and capital investment decisions. Some Trusts will benefit as a result of this process but some will not, and the spontaneous emergence of a suitable solution to the problem is highly unlikely. Given the centrality of medical manpower to the maintenance of a viable NHS, it is inevitable that the planning and coordination of services which are key to postgraduate training will have to be enforced across Trusts by an alliance of Postgraduate Deans, Regional Training Committees and Health Authorities.

However, although the planning of the local distribution of NHS provision is likely to re-emerge as an important feature of bureaucratic power, the attempt to drive this activity through the introduction of the commissioner–provider division and the new Health Authority function of needs identification has largely failed. Health Authorities were given the responsibility for making public choices about the disposal of finite health care resources. That they have struggled to do so in a manner regarded as legitimate by their local populations is to be expected: the hegemony of the welfare state does not accept that rights can be prioritised: that one individual's health care rights are more important, or less important, than another's. Hence when clear choices have been made by commissioning agencies, as in the Child B case (Chadda, 1995), for example, public outrage has been easily aroused. In the early days of the 1991 reforms it was assumed that rational procedures informed by epidemiological and/or economistic evidence could be used to determine and legitimate priorities along bureaucratically reproducible lines such as those used in the Oregon experiment in the United States. But this has proved to be neither technically nor politically feasible.

Equally, politicians have shown themselves reluctant to commit political *hara-kiri* by establishing national rationing criteria which would inevitably challenge the founding values of the NHS. Instead they have continued to insist that the allocative conundrum should be resolved at the local level. Their difficulty is that the Beveridge model of state health care, unlike the Bismarck model, does not allow them to distance themselves from their duty to their citizens but neither can they resolve the political problem this creates. As Taylor-Gooby observes:

> In a social insurance system the central problem is how to control medical costs; in state-controlled systems, it is whether funding is adequate and how to handle the problems of deciding priorities and deal with waiting lists and rationing measures. (Taylor-Gooby, 1996: 217)

With Health Authority bureaucrats and national politicians both unable to deal publicly with the demand–supply mismatch, the issue has had to be resolved, as previously, at the level of the provider organisations by managers and doctors.

The logic of the 1991 reforms was that Trust managers would use their new found operational freedoms to insist that clinicians form part of the corporate effort to fulfil the contractual agreements with commissioning agencies and, following the introduction of the

Patient's Charter, the Charter's targets. Pursuing this logic, it was assumed that doctors would adjust their clinical decision-making and their waiting lists (the primary rationing mechanism) to suit the needs of their employing organisation. If implemented, such a shift would have meant a reduction in the doctors' clinical and political autonomy and an enhancement of managerial power. In the control-of-demand game, the logic meant that the commissioners would define the populations's health care needs, managers would arrange for the services to meet those needs, and doctors would ensure that the patients they saw and the conditions they treated in the provision of those services (the met demand) equalled the needs identified by the commissioners. How has the balance of power between managers and doctors been redefined in practice?

Klein has speculated that the new-model NHS may have strengthened awareness of an inter-dependence between managers and clinicians:

> If managers cannot mobilise the support of clinicians for their strategies, they are unlikely to succeed in achieving the targets on which the renewal of their contracts depends; they may even indeed be forced out of office if they antagonise medical staff. Conversely, however, clinicians will not attract the resources they need to develop their services if they block or subvert managers: they need efficient, active management for survival. (Klein, 1995: 324)

New forms of mutual accommodation, he argues, may therefore have developed as a result. Whilst accepting that managers need clinicians and clinicians need managers, however, there is a further question of which of the partners in this relationship is likely to be the dominant one. In addressing this issue it is important to retain a grasp on the basis of group power in the NHS and not to be seduced into attaching undue significance into the changing kaleidescope of organisational forms which the groups inhabit.

At one level it would seem that clinicians have allowed managers to exercise influence in the key rationing territory of waiting lists. It is undoubtedly the case that in response to urgings from managers about the penalties that lie in store for non-compliance, waiting lists have been dramatically reduced. But is this an indicator of increased managerial power or an illustration of how the medical profession can adapt its rationing role in order to retain both control of the rationing function and the personal and professional benefits that accrue from its operation? It will be remembered from Chapter 3 that waiting lists are a mechanism for providing consultants with status (longer waiting lists equals demand for valued service) and private income (diversion of waiting list patients into the private practice). At present the maximum waiting list time is 18 months and this is quite sufficient for the lists to continue to perform their traditional function on behalf of consultants as well as meeting managers' needs. So it can be argued that clinicians have accommodated managers at no cost to themselves.

Managers still have very few direct levers of control that they can use to direct clinicians' activity. They can badger, argue and perhaps persuade but they have no ultimate sanction: consultants cannot be sacked unless they are deserted by their professional colleagues. Nor do managers have any template against which to measure clinicians' activity and performance: the much vaunted job plans for clinicians have rarely moved beyond the cosmetic adjustments required to demonstrate consistency with the relevant NHSE circular; medical audit remains firmly within medicine's professional orbit; and management's putative influence over the new, local distinction awards for consultants has yet to be demonstrated in practice. On the other side of the coin, managers are very vulnerable to clinician pressure. A vote of no confidence in a manager by consultants is a clear signal that their employment with a particular Trust is about to be terminated.

At the same time, the ability of managers to develop their power base in Trusts has been severely constrained by the ability of the bureaucrats to circumscribe Trust freedoms. Despite the promises of the reforms, the devolution of operational control has not been accompanied by a diminution of the bureaucratic jungle; in fact, quite the opposite. It has grown and it has prospered in the intense political sunlight of the Health Service presenting managers with a dense undergrowth of accountability foliage within which they are obliged to move. Managers may have been born free in *Working for Patients* but everywhere in the NHS they are in chains.

Whether they survive as a power group in the NHS depends very much on the direction taken by the ruling class: the medical profession. The politicians have already made it clear that they no longer see managers as the heroic figures of the NHS, battling to impose order on recalcitrant clinicians. As the inability of the organisational changes of 1991 to make any dent in the underlying problem of excess demand has become apparent, so the politicians have been obliged to return to their historic concordat with the medical profession as the vehicle for the primary political task of rationing. As a consequence, managers have found themselves sidelined and scapegoated by politicians of all parties as a cause of cost inflation in the Health Service. One unequivocal indicator of their fall from favour was the 1995 edict by the Secretary of State, Steven Dorrell, that management costs should be reduced by 5 per cent. At the level of popular rhetoric (an increasingly significant form of symbolic exchange in the NHS and its political environs), this move found expression in the Minister's preference for 'less grey suits and more white coats'.

The signs are that the medical profession has learnt its lesson from the short, sharp, shock of the 1989 Review and its aftermath. There the profession was neglected, cold-shouldered and marginalised. Now its traditional value to the NHS and to the state is being re-emphasised and the profession is taking steps to put its own house in order. As a result, it is probable as Klein observes, that 'the most important consequence of the NHS reforms may thus be not so much that they changed the balance of power between clinicians and managers but that they prompted the medical profession to take pre-emptive action to prevent such a shift taking place' (*ibid.*: 325). At the national level, this action involves the medical elites of the Royal Colleges, General Medical Council (GMC) and British Medical Association (BMA) improving the efficiency with which they manage their own territory in terms of training, professional standards and career progress. To do this they will have both to refine their own bureaucracies and to engage much more fully with the bureaucracy of the NHS. If a substantial alliance between medicine's national bodies and parts of the NHS bureaucracy is engineered (for example, through a more direct management role for the Postgraduate Dean in postgraduate training), then it is likely to be at the expense of the clinical and political autonomy of the individual clinician. Medicine as a collectivity will maintain its autonomy but its members will be obliged to submit to a more rigorous regime of professional monitoring.

At the local level, much depends on the willingness of clinicians to assume a more active management role. Their power will be enhanced if they do but will not be diminished if they do not. In career terms, there are few incentives and clear disincentives for consultants to take up the management cudgels. Management experience is not a factor in distinction awards (apart from the small local awards) and for clinical directors there is rarely a significant remuneration for their pains to compensate them for the loss of private practice and income which is frequently a consequence of the time commitment involved. More generally, medicine's professional culture does not as yet place much value on the management activity and, indeed, it is seen by some as antithetical to the exercise of clinical freedom. In sum, it is likely that clinicians will do sufficient management to protect their professional patch at the clinical directorate level but will not attempt to take over the demanding quasi-political role of senior management in the Trusts.

For reasons of professional inertia and clinician convenience, managers will therefore survive as a power group in the NHS; tolerated by the doctors, monitored by the bureaucrats, and blamed by the politicians. In practice, their role will continue to be the necessary one of synthesizing and balancing the numerous political pressures that congregate at the door of the Trusts, but they have yet to make political capital out of this necessity.

Although the reforms have had the effect of reinforcing the traditional divisions within medicine between the specialists in the hospitals and the general practitioners in primary care, this has not served to diminish medicine's overall power. What it has achieved is a new balance of power across the internal division. GP Fundholders now have the power of the purse as a counter-balance to the status differential between themselves and specialists – and this they will not relinquish easily. Command of the financial resources for secondary care has also caused Fundholders to think more seriously about the appropriateness of their patterns of referrals to consultants who, in turn, have to be sensitive to signicant shifts in the referrals they receive since these are the source of their private practice business.

The right of consultants to earn substantial sums from their private practice is a reflection of their influential position in the NHS and the flexible contractual arrangements which they negotiated in 1948 when the Health Service was founded. In a very real sense, the privileged position of medicine within the NHS is buttressed by its dominant position in the private sector. Equally, its key function in both public and private sectors means that a commitment to change in one will impact on its involvment in the other. As Laing and Buisson observe, within the private health care sector consultants:

> have a virtual monopoly of private practice because of the professionally established referral chain from GPs to consultants, because of professional rules which prevent specialists from advertising direct to the public and because of private medical insurance rules which, with a few exceptions restrict reimbursement to treatment provided by specialists who have attained

consultant status. (Laing and Buisson, 1995: A119)

It is not a position which, as a body, they would be happy to relinquish. 71 per cent of consultants engage in private practice and in 1992 mean and median gross private practice earnings were £33 000 and £24 000 respectively (*ibid.*). In 1993 The Monopolies and Mergers Commission determined that a 'complex monopoly' exists in the supply of private medical services, consisting of those consultants who set their fees close to the BMA guidelines (Monopolies and Mergers Commission, 1993). Two years later the BMA agreed to discontinue the publication of the guidelines, thus eliminating the upward pressure on consultant fees, but it is doubtful whether this will undermine the consultants' dominant position in the private market.

Given the consultants' grip on the supply of patients and expertise to the private sector, there is a theoretical overlap of interest between private sector provider managers who wish to contain or reduce their staffing costs and NHS Trust managers who wish to make their consultants more accountable. Both would welcome a reduction in consultant power. Neither is likely to get it because managers are divided by their competition for patients and dependent upon the medical profession to supply them.

Conclusions

There is a surreal quality to the NHS reforms of the 1990s. In an organisational sense they were the most significant since 1948, introducing new structures, new processes and a new language of official intercourse. Founded on the functional divide between commissioners and providers they ushered into being a new contract culture where targets are set, costs identified and performance measured. Transparency has become the norm, not only in terms of the cost-effective use of resources under the watchful eye of the Audit Commission, but also in terms of more general aspects of governance such as accountability to the patient and to the local community.

But in a fundamental political sense, these same changes are an illusion, a theatre of intense activity where the scene shifting is dramatic but the relative power positions of the actors on the stage alters but little. Yet the actors – the politicians, the bureaucrats, the managers and the doctors – must not only engage to play out their NHS roles given the balance of power between them, they must also continue to make their respective contributions to the underlying political problem of the mismatch between citizen demand and health care supply. To the extent that the new policy framework allows them to do so, their power will increase; to the extent that it does not, their power will diminish.

What has been clearly shown by the reforms is that changes in the organisation of the supply side of the political equation can contribute little to the amelioration of the problem. Improved efficiency in the delivery of state health care, the basic tenet of the reforms, does not impact on the demand–supply mismatch in any significant sense because of the elasticity of the demand. In the absence of a restrictive definition of health care rights and of any mechanism to attribute a cost to expressed demand, that elasticity is infinite and, indeed, is highly sensitive to changes in supply. More supply means more health care opportunities which, in turn, stimulate more demand.

Whilst welfare state values maintain their hegemony and exclude public recognition that it is a rights-driven, demand-side problem, the political parties will remain impotent to address the issue and will be obliged, as ever, to rely on the beneficence of the medical profession. But how long the doctors are able to stem the tide of citizen expectation is questionable. Rising levels of education, alternative sources of information, and evidence of conflicting medical views have served to undermine medicine's authority and, therefore, its political efficacy. Until the state is able to escape its self-made ideological prison and confront its citizens' expectations, its only option is recognise the extent of its exposure and shore up the medical profession.

References

Aggleton P. and Chalmers H. (1986) *Nursing Models and the Nursing Process*, Basingstoke, Macmillan.

Allen I. (1988) *Doctors and Their Careers*, London, Policy Studies Institute.

Allen I. (1994) *Doctors and Their Careers. A New Generation*, London, Policy Studies Institute.

Allsop J. (1995) *Health Policy and the NHS. Towards 2000*, London, Longman.

Anderson T.F. and Mooney G. (eds) (1990) *The Challenges of Medical Practice Variations*, Basingstoke, Macmillan.

Appleby J. (1995) 'RAWP: weighting for a chance', *Health Service Journal*, 13 July: 34–5.

Armstrong D., Britten N. and Grace J. (1988) 'Measuring general practitioners referrals: patient workload and list size', *Journal of the Royal College of General Practitioners*, **38**: 494–7.

Armstrong D., Fry J. and Armstrong P. (1991) 'Doctors perceptions of pressure from patients for referral', *British Medical Journal*, **302**: 1186–8.

Ascher K. (1987) *The Politics of Privatisation: Contracting Out Public Services*, Basingstoke, Macmillan.

Ashburner L. and Cairncross L. (1992) 'Just trust in us', *Health Service Journal*, 14 May: 20–2.

Audit Commission (1986) *Making A Reality of Community Care*, London, HMSO.

Audit Commission (1989) 'Developing community care for people with a mental illness', *Hansard*, 19 November 1991, written answer, Mentally Ill People.

Audit Commission (1991) *The Virtue of Patients: Making Best Use of Ward Nursing Resources*, London, HMSO.

Audit Commission (1992a) *Homeward Bound, A New Course for Community Health*, London, HMSO.

Audit Commission (1992b) *Community Care: Managing the Cascade of Change*, London, HMSO.
Audit Commission (1992c) *The Community Revolution: Personal Social Services and Community Care*, London, HMSO.
Audit Commission (1993) *Practice Makes Perfect: The Role of the Family Health Service Authority*, London, HMSO.
Audit Commission (1994a) *Trusting in the Future*, London, HMSO.
Audit Commission (1994b) *Protecting the Public Purse 2*, London, HMSO.
Audit Commission (1994c) *Finding A Place. A Review of Mental Health Services for Adults*, London, HMSO.
Audit Commission (1995a) *Taken on Board – Corporate Governance in the NHS. Developing the Role of Non-executive Directors*, London, HMSO.
Audit Commission (1995b) *A Price on their Heads – Measuring Management Costs in NHS Trusts*, London, HMSO.
Audit Commission (1995c) *Briefing on GP Fundholding*, London, HMSO.
Audit Commission (1996a) *What the Doctor Ordered. A Study of GP Fundholders in England and Wales*, London, HMSO.
Audit Commission (1996b) *Balancing the Care Equation: Progress with Community Care*, London, HMSO.
Auplish S. and Shires L. (1994) 'Who goes where', *Health Service Journal*, 15 September: 24–5.
Balarajan R. (1990) *Social Deprivation and Age Adjustment Ratios for South West Thames Region*, Guildford, Epidemiology and Public Health Research Unit, Guildford, Surrey University.
Barker P. (1990) 'The Leicester experience', *Health Service Journal*, 27 September: 9.
Baroness Macfarlane of Llandaff and Castledine G. (1982) *A Guide to the Practice of Nursing Using the Nursing Process*, London, C.V. Mosby.
Bartlett W. (1991) *Privatisation and Quasi-Markets*, DQM7, Bristol, School for Advanced Urban Studies, University of Bristol.
Bartlett W. and Le Grand J. (1993) 'The theory of quasi-markets' in Le Grand J. and Bartlett W. (eds) *Quasi-Markets and Social Policy*, London, Macmillan.
Beecham L. (1990) 'Reservations on nurse prescribing', *British Medical Journal*, **300**: 1275–6.
Beecham L. (1994) 'Managers will have more say in merit awards', *British Medical Journal*, **309**: 1187–8.
Bellamy R. (1993) 'Citizenship and rights' in Bellamy R. (ed.) *Theories and Concepts of Politics*, Manchester, Manchester University Press.

Biggs J. (1994) 'Postgraduate medical education in the NHS; increasing effort and impact through 25 years', *Health Trends*, **26**(1): 5–10.

Bliss A. and Cohen E. (eds) (1977) *The New Health Professionals: Nurse Practitioners and Physician Assistants*, Colorado, Aspen.

Brearley S. (1994) 'The failure of consultant expansion', *British Medical Journal*, **309**: 1245–6.

Breen D. (1991) 'Setting priorities: a framework for the assessment of health care priorities', *Health Bulletin*, **49**(1): 34–9.

Brenton M. (1985) *The Voluntary Sector in British Social Services*, London, Longman.

Briggs A. (1961) 'The welfare state in historical perspective', *European Journal of Sociology*, **2**: 221–58.

Bright J. (1985) *A Critique of Methods for Determining Nursing Staffing Levels in Hospitals,* DHSS Operational Research Service, London, DHSS.

British Association of Medical Managers, British Medical Association, Institute of Health Service Management, Royal College of Nursing (1993) *Managing Clinical Services: A Consensus Statement of Principles for Effective Clinical Management*, London, IHSM.

British Medical Association (1970) *Health Service Financing*, London, BMA.

British Medical Association (1992) *Priorities for Community Care: A British Medical Association Report*, London, BMA.

British Medical Association (1995a) *Survey of the Impact of the Implementation of the Community Care Reforms*, London, BMA.

British Medical Association (1995b) *Survey of the Impact of the Implementation of the Community Care Reforms: Psychiatrists and Geriatricians*, London, BMA.

British Medical Association Central Consultants and Specialists Committee (1990) *Guidance on Clinical Directorates*, London, BMA.

British Medical Journal (1994) 'General Medical Council says it will watch curriculum reforms', *British Medical Journal*, editorial, **308**(5): 361.

British Medical Journal and General Medical Services Committee (1992) *The Future of General Practice*, London, British Medical Journal Publishing Group.

Browning D. (1992) 'Getting ready for change', *British Medical Journal*, **305**: 1415–18.

Buchan J. (1992) 'Nurse manpower planning: role, rationale and relevance' in Robinson J., Gray A. and Elkan R. (eds) *Policy Issues in Nursing*, Buckingham, Open University Press, pp. 38–51.

Butland G. (1993) 'Commissioning for quality', *British Medical Journal*, **306**: 251–2.

Butler J. (1992) *Patients, Policies and Politics,* Buckingham, Open University Press.

Caine N. (1993) 'Heart to heart: transplant clinicians assistants have come to play a vital role', *Health Service Journal*, **103**(5370): 21–4.

Calman K. (1994a) 'The profession of medicine', *British Medical Journal*, **309**: 1140–3.

Calman K. (1994b) *Continuing Medical Education*, consultation paper, London, DoH.

Calnan M., Cant S. and Gabe J. (1993) *Going Private: Why People Pay for their Health Care*, Buckingham, Open University Press.

Campling E.A., Devlin H.B., Hoile R.W. and Lunn J.N. (1992) *The Report of the National Confidential Enquiry into Perioperative Deaths 1990*, London, National Confidential Enquiry into Perioperative Deaths.

Carey T., Garrett, A., Jackman, C. *et al.* (1995) 'The outcomes and costs of care for acute low back pain among patients seen by primary care practitioners, chiropractors, and orthopaedic surgeons', *New England Journal of Medicine*, **333**: 913–7.

Carpenter M. (1977) 'The new managerialism and professionalism in nursing' in Stacey M., Reid M. and Heath C. (eds) *Health and the Division of Labour*, Beckenham, Croom Helm.

Carr-Hill R. and Sheldon T. (1992) 'Rationality and the use of formulae in the allocation of resources to health care', *Journal of Public Health Medicine*, **14**(2): 117–26.

Catford J.C. (1991) 'Health targets', *British Medical Journal*, **302**: 980–1.

Central Statistical Office (1993) *Social Trends*, London, HMSO.

Central Statistical Office (1994) *Social Trends*, London, HMSO.

Central Statistical Office (1996) *Social Trends*, London, HMSO.

Centre for Health Economics (1995) *Equality in Primary Care*, Discussion Paper 141, University of York.

Chadda D. (1993) 'The new deal', *Health Service Journal*, 2 September: 12.

Chadda D. (1994) 'What a performance' *Health Service Journal*, 15 September: 11.

Chadda D. (1995) 'Child B health commission would fund evaluated care', *Health Service Journal*, 24 August: 4.

Chancellor of the Exchequer, Secretary of State for Social Security, President of The Board of Trade, Secretary of State For Health, Secretary of State for Northern Ireland, Secretary of State for Scotland, Secretary of State for Wales (1996) *A New Partnership in Old Age*, Cm 3242, London, HMSO.

Chant A.D.B. (1984) 'National Health Service: practising doctors should not manage', *Lancet*, **1**(8391): 1398.

Chantler C. (1990) 'Managerial reform in a London hospital' in Carle N. (ed.) *Managing for Health Result*, London, King Edward's Hospital Fund for London, pp. 74–85.

Charney M.C., Lewis P.A. and Farrow S.C. (1989) 'Choosing who should not be treated in the National Health Service', *Social Science and Medicine*, **28**: 1331–8.

Chief Nursing Officers for England, Wales, Scotland and Northern Ireland (1993) *The Challenges for Nursing and Midwifery in the 21st century,* The Heathrow Debate, London, DoH.

Clark R.W. and Gray C. (1994) 'Options for change in the National Health Service consultant contract', *British Medical Journal*, **309**: 528–30.

Cochrane M., Ham C., Heginbotham C. and Smith R. (1991) 'Rationing: at the cutting edge', *British Medical Journal*, **303**(6809): 1039–42.

Committee on Nursing (1972) *Report of the Committee on Nursing*, (Chair: Professor A. Briggs) Cmnd 5115, London, HMSO.

Community Care Support Force (1992) *Implementing Community Care: Delivering the Key Tasks. A Guide for All Health Authorities*, London, Price Waterhouse.

Connolly M. (1991) 'Hail the Belfast pioneers', *Health Service Journal*, 7 February, 22–3.

Cooper M.H. (1975) *Rationing Health Care*, London, Croom Helm.

Coopers and Lybrand (1988) *Integrated Analysis for the Review of RAWP*, London, Coopers and Lybrand.

Coulter A. (1995a) 'Shifting the balance from secondary to primary care', *British Medical Journal*, **311**: 1447–8.

Coulter A. (1995b) 'Evaluating general practitioner fundholding in the UK', *European Journal of Public Health*, **5**: 233–9.

Coulter A. and Bradlow J. (1993) 'Effect of NHS reforms on general practitioner referral patterns', *British Medical Journal*, **306**: 433–7.

Culyer A. (1994) *Supporting Research and Development in the NHS*, London, HMSO.

Cummins R., Jarman B. and White P. (1981) 'Do general practitioners have different referral thresholds?' *Journal of the Royal College of General Practitioners*, **37**: 350–3.

Day M. (1995) 'Practitioners make perfect', *Nursing Times*, **91**(15): 22.

Day P. (1992) 'Accountability', paper for the Rowntree Symposium, University of Birmingham, 19–20 November.

Delamothe T. (1992) 'Getting rational over rationing', *British Medical Journal*, **305**: 1240–1.

Delamothe T. (1994) *Outcomes into Clinical Practice*, London, British Medical Journal Publishing Group.

Department of Health (1989a) *Working for Patients*, Cm 555, London, HMSO.

Department of Health (1989b) *NHS Consultants: Appointments, Contracts and Distinction Awards*, Working for Patients, Working Paper 7, London, HMSO.

Department of Health (1989c) *Education and Training*, Working for Patients, Working Paper 10, London, HMSO.

Department of Health (1989d) *Self-governing Hospitals*, Working for Patients, Working Paper 1, London, HMSO.

Department of Health (1989e) *Implications for Family Practitioner Committees*, Working for Patients, Working Paper 8, London, HMSO.

Department of Health (1989f) *Caring for People: Community Care in the Next Decade and Beyond*, Cm 849, London, HMSO.

Department of Health (1989g) *Indicative Prescribing Budgets for General Practitioners*, Working for Patients, Working Paper 4, London, HMSO.

Department of Health (1989h) *Practice Budgets for General Medical Practitioners*, Working for Patients, Working Paper 3, London, HMSO.

Department of Health (1990a) *Developing Districts*, London, HMSO.

Department of Health (1990b) *Disciplinary Procedures for Hospital and Community Medical and Dental Staff*, HC(90)9, London, DoH.

Department of Health (1990c) *Community Care in the Next Decade and Beyond: Policy Guidance*, London, HMSO.

Department of Health (1991) *The Health of the Nation*, Consultative Document, London, DoH, (Green Paper).

Department of Health (1992a) *The Patient's Charter*, London, HMSO.

Department of Health (1992b) *The Health of the Nation, A Strategy for Health in England*, Cm 1986, London, HMSO, (White Paper).

Department of Health (1992c) *The Health of the Nation: Specification of National Indicators*, London, DoH.

Department of Health (1993a) *Managing the New NHS, A Background Document*, London, DoH.

Department of Health (1993b) *One Year On... A Report on Progress on the Health of the Nation*, London, DoH.

Department of Health (1993c) *Changing Childbirth*, Expert Maternity Group, London, HMSO.

Department of Health (1994a) *Being Heard,* The Report of the Review Committee on NHS Procedures (Chair: Professor A. Wilson), London, DoH.

Department of Health (1994b) *Review of the Wider Department of Health*, London, DoH.

Department of Health (1994c) *Implementing Caring for People. The Role of the GP and Primary Health Care Team*, London, DoH.

Department of Health (1995a) *Statement of Responsibilities and Accountabilities*, London, DoH.

Department of Health (1995b) *The Patient's Charter and You*, London, DoH.

Department of Health (1995c) *Fit for the Future, Second Progress Report on the Health of the Nation*, London, DoH.

Department of Health (1995d) *Government Response to the First Report from the Health Committee, Session 1994–95, Priority Setting in the NHS: Purchasing*, Cm 2826, London, HMSO.

Department of Health (1995e) *NHS Responsibilities for Meeting Continuing Care Needs*, HSG(95)8 and LAC(95)5, London, DoH.

Department of Health (1995f) *Health and Personal Social Services Statistics for England*, London, HMSO.

Department of Health (1996a) *The Spectrum of Care. Local Services for People with Mental Health Problems*, Health of the Nation, London, DoH.

Department of Health (1996b) *Building Bridges. A Guide to Arrangements for Inter-Agency Working for the Care and Protection of Severely Mentally Ill People*, London, DoH.

Department of Health (1996c) *Press Release* 96/188, 3 June.

Department of Health (1997) *Developing Partnerships in Mental Health*, Cm 3555, London, HMSO.

Department of Health and Department of the Environment (1994) *Framework for Local Community Care Charters in England*, HSG(94)24 and LAC(94)47, London, DoH.

Department of Health and Department of the Environment (1995) *New Guidance on Local Authority Community Care Plans*, LAC(95)19, London, DoH.

Department of Health and Social Security (1971) *Better Services for the Mentally Handicapped*, London, HMSO.

Department of Health and Social Security (1972) *Management Arrangements for the Reorganised Health Service*, London, HMSO.

Department of Health and Social Security (1975) *Better Services for the Mentally Ill*, London, HMSO.

Department of Health and Social Security (1976) *Priorities for the Health and Personal Social Services*, London, HMSO.

Department of Health and Social Security (1977) *The Extending Role of the Clinical Nurse – Legal Implications and Training Requirements*, HC(77)22, London, DHSS.

Department of Health and Social Security (1981) *Care in Action: A Handbook of Policies and Priorities for the Health and Personal Social Services in England*, London, HMSO.

Department of Health and Social Security (1982) *Prevention of Harm to Patients Resulting from Physical or Mental Disability of Hospital or Community Medical or Dental Staff*, HC(82)13, London, DHSS.

Department of Health and Social Security (1983a) *NHS Management Inquiry*, Griffith's Report, London, HMSO.

Department of Health and Social Security (1983b) *Medical Act 1983*, London, HMSO.

Department of Health and Social Security (1986a) *Neighbourhood Nursing: A Focus for Care,* A Report of the Community Nursing Review in England (Chair: Julia Cumberlege), London, HMSO.

Department of Health and Social Security (1986b) *Health Services Management: Resource Management (Management Budgeting) in Health Authorities*, Circular HN(86)34, London, HMSO.

Department of Health and Social Security (1987a) *Promoting Better Health. The Government's Programme for Improving Primary Health Care*, Cm 249, London, HMSO.

Department of Health and Social Security (1987b) Steering group for implementation on behalf of the UK Health Departments, the Joint Consultants Committee, and chairmen of Regional Health Authorities, *Achieving a Balance: Plan for Action*, London, DHSS.

Department of Health and Social Security (1988) Committee of inquiry into the future development of the public health function, *Public Health in England*, Cm 289, London, HMSO (Acheson report).

Department of Health, Social Services Inspectorate and Scottish Office Social Work Services Group (1991) *Care Management and Assessment*: Managers' Guide, London, DoH.

Dixon J. and Glennerster H. (1995) 'What do we know about fundholding in general practice?', *British Medical Journal*, **311**: 727–30.

Dixon J. and Welch H.G. (1991) 'Priority setting: lessons from Oregon', *Lancet*, **337**: 890–4.

Dobson J. (1992) 'Wall demands DoH guidance on cash for community care', *Health Service Journal*, 8 October: 7.

Dobson J. (1993) 'Fingers crossed', *Health Service Journal*, 18 February: 13.

Donaldson L. (1995) 'The listening blank', *Health Service Journal*, 21 September, 22–3.

Donaldson L.J. (1994a) 'Doctors with problems in the NHS workforce', *British Medical Journal*, **308**: 1277–82.

Donaldson L.J. (1994b) 'Sick doctors: a responsibility to act', *British Medical Journal*, **309**: 557–8.

Donaldson C. and Farrar S. (1991) *Needs Assessment: Developing an Economic Approach*, Health Education Research Unit Discussion Paper, York, University of York.

Donaldson C. and Mooney G. (1991) 'Needs assessment, priority setting, and contracts for health care: an economic view', *British Medical Journal*, **303**: 1529–30.

Dowie R. (1987) *Postgraduate Medical Education and Training: The System in England and Wales*, London, King Edward's Hospital Fund for London.

Dowling S. and Barrett S. (1992) *Doctors in the Making. The Experience of the Pre-registration Year*, Bristol, School for Advanced Urban Studies.

Dowling S., Martin R., Skidmore P. *et al.* (1996) 'Nurses taking on junior doctors work: a confusion of accountability', *British Medical Journal*, **312**: 1211–14.

Dudley N.J. and Burns E. (1992) 'The influence of age on policies for admission and thrombolysis in coronary care units in the UK', *Age and Ageing*, **21**: 95–8.

Dymond D.S. and Lim R. (1994) 'Defining "emergency" and "urgency": the domino effect', *Journal of the Royal College of Physicians of London*, **28**(4): 286–7.

Elston M.A. (1991) 'The politics of professional power: medicine in a changing health service' in Gabe J., Calnan M. and Bury M. (eds) *The Sociology of the Health Service*, London, Routledge: Ch. 3.

Elwell H. (1986) *NHS, The Road to Recovery*, London, Centre for Policy Studies.

English National Board for Nursing, Midwifery and Health Visiting (1993) *Framework for Continuing Professional Education and Higher Award for Nurses, Midwives and Health Visitors*, London, ENB.

English National Board for Nursing, Midwifery and Health Visiting (1995) *Annual Report*, London, ENB.

Enthoven A.C. (1985) *Reflections on the Management of the National Health Service*, London, Nuffield Provincial Hospitals Trust.

Eskin F. and Bull A. (1991) 'Squaring a difficult circle', *Health Service Journal*, 10 January: 16–17.

Evers A. (1993) 'The welfare mix approach; understanding the pluralism of welfare systems' in Evers A. and Svetlik I. (eds)

Balancing Pluralism: New Welfare Mixes in Care for the Elderly, Aldershot, Avery.

Ewart I. (1991) 'A family matter', *Health Service Journal*, 9 May: 18–20.

Ferguson B. and Ryder S. (1991) *The Future of the DHA: Assessing Needs for Services and Setting Priorities*, York Health Economics Consortium, University of York.

Ferlie E. and Ashburner L. (1993) 'Moves and shakers', *Health Service Journal*, 18 November: 24–6.

Ferlie E., Ashburner L. and Fitzgerald L. (1993) *Board Teams – Roles and Relationships*, Research for Action Paper 10, Bristol, NHS Training Directorate.

Ferlie E., Challis D. and Davies B. (1989) *Efficiency – Improving Innovations in the Social Care of the Elderly*, Aldershot, Gower.

Fitzgerald L. (1991a) 'Made to measure', *Health Service Journal*, 31 October: 24–5.

Fitzgerald L. (1991b) 'This year's model', *Health Service Journal*, 7 November: 24–5.

Ford R. and Sathyamoorthy G. (1996) 'Team games', *Health Service Journal*, 27 June: 32–3.

Foster A. (1991) *FHSAs: Today's and Tomorrow's Priorities*, Leeds, NHSME.

Garbett R. (1996) 'The growth of nurse-led care', *Nursing Times*, **92**(1): 29.

General Medical Council (1993) *Professional Conduct and Discipline: Fitness to Practice*, London, GMC.

General Medical Council (1994) *Annual Report*, London, GMC.

General Medical Council, Education Committee (1987) *Recommendations on the Training of Specialists*, London, GMC.

Gladstone D. (1992) *Opening Up the Medical Monopoly*, London, Adam Smith Institute.

Glennerster H., Matsaganis M. and Owens P. (1992) *A Foothold for Fundholding*, London, King's Fund Institute.

Glennerster H., Matsaganis M. and Owens P. (1994) *Implementing GP Fundholding*, Buckingham, Open University Press.

Goldsmith M. and Willetts D. (1988) *Managed Health Care: A New System for a Better Health Service*, London, Centre for Policy Studies.

Goss S. and Kent C. (1995) *Health and Housing: Working Together?*, Bristol, The Policy Press/Joseph Rowntree.

Graffy J.P. and Williams J. (1994) 'Purchasing for all: an alternative to fundholding', *British Medical Journal*, **308**: 391–4.

Graineer L. (1995) 'Evaluating pre-operative care', *Nursing Times*, **91**(15): 31–2.

Green D. (1986) *Challenge to the NHS*, Hobart Paperback no. 23, London, Institute of Economic Affairs.

Green D. (1988) *Everyone A Private Patient*, Hobart Paperback no. 27, London, Institute of Economic Affairs.

Green D.G., Neuberger J., Lord Young of Dartington and Burstall M.L. (1990) *The NHS Reforms: Whatever Happened to Consumer Choice?* London, Institute of Economic Affairs, Health and Welfare Unit.

Greenhalgh and Co. (1994) *The Interface Between Junior Doctors and Nurses: A Research Study for the Department of Health*, London, Greenhalgh and Co.

Greer P. (1994) *Transforming Central Government: The Next Steps Initiative*, Milton Keynes, Open University Press.

Griffith B., Iliffe S. and Rayner G. (1981) *Banking on Sickness*, London: Lawrence & Wishart.

Griffiths P. and Evans A. (1995) *Evaluation of a Nursing-led In-patient Service. An Interim Report*, London, King's Fund Centre.

Griffiths Sir Roy (1988) *Community Care: An Agenda for Action*, London, HMSO.

Grosney M. and Tallis R. (1991) 'The burden of chronic illness in local authority residential homes for the elderly', *Health Trends*, **22**(4): 153–7.

Grossman J.H. (1990) 'Physicians as managers in hospitals' in Costain D. (ed.) *The Future of Acute Services: Doctors as Managers*, London, King's Fund Centre for Health Services Development.

Gulland A. (1996) 'Private finance, public nightmare', *BMA News Review*, January: 18–19.

Hadley R. and Hatch S. (1981) *Social Welfare and the Failure of the State: Centralised Social Services and Participatory Alternatives*, London, Allen & Unwin.

Hadley T. (1996) 'Splitting the difference', *Health Service Journal*, 11 April, 21.

Hadorn D.C. (1991) 'The role of public values in setting health care priorities', *Social Science and Medicine*, **32**(7): 773–81.

Halper T. (1989) *The Misfortunes of Others: End-stage Renal Disease in the UK*, Cambridge, Cambridge University Press.

Ham C. (1985) *Health Policy in Britain*, Basingstoke, Macmillan Education.

Ham C. and Heginbotham C. (1991a) 'How to make a future champion', *Health Service Journal*, 25 July.

Ham C. and Heginbotham C. (1991b) *Purchasing Together*, London, King's Fund College Paper.

Hann M. (1993) 'The training cash web unravelled', *BMA News Review*, October: 22–3.

Hann M. (1994a) 'Training the trainers', *BMA News Review*, May: 22.
Hann M. (1994b) 'Trusts struggle to meet 56-hour target, *BMA News Review*, December: 16.
Hannay D.R. (1993) 'Primary care and public health', *British Medical Journal*, **307**: 516–17.
Hardy B., Wistow G. and Rhodes R.A.W. (1990) 'Policy networks and the implementation of community care policy for people with mental handicaps', *Journal of Social Policy*, **19**(2): 141–68.
Harrison S. (1988) *Managing the Health Service: Shifting the Frontier*, London: Chapman & Hall.
Harrison S. and Pollitt C. (1994) *Controlling Health Professionals: The Future of Work and Organisation in the NHS*, Buckingham, Open University Press.
Harrison S., Hunter D., Marnoch G. and Pollitt C.J. (1989) *The Impact of General Management in the NHS*, Leeds, Nuffield Institute.
Harrison S., Hunter D.J. and Marnoch G. (1992) *Just Managing: Power and Culture in the NHS*, Leeds, Nuffield Institute.
Hart C. (1994) *Behind the Mask. Nurses, Their Unions and Nursing Policy*, London, Baillière Tindall.
Hatch S. and Mocroft I. (1983) *Components of Welfare*, London, Bedford Square Press.
Haug M. (1973) 'Deprofessionalisation: an alternative hypothesis for the future', *Sociological Review Monograph*, **20**: 195–211.
Haug M. (1988) 'A re-examination of the hypothesis of deprofessionalisation', *The Millbank Quarterly*, **66**(suppl. 2): 48–56.
Healthcare 2000 (1995) *UK Health and Healthcare Services. Challenges and Policy Options,* London, King's Fund Policy Institute.
Health Committee of the House of Commons (1993) *Community Care: Funding from April 1993*, Third Report, Session 1992–93, London, HMSO.
Health Committee of the House of Commons (1995a) *Priority Setting in the NHS: Purchasing*, First Report, vol. I, Session 1994–95, HC 134–1, London, HMSO.
Health Committee of the House of Commons (1995b) *Long-term Care: NHS Responsibilities for Meeting Continuing Care Needs*, First Report, vol. I, Session 1995–96, HC19–I, London, HMSO.
Health Committee of the House of Commons (1989) *General Practice in the National Health Service, The 1990 Contract*, London, Department of Health.
Health Service Journal (1993) 'Rocking chairs', *Health Service Journal*, 25 March: 17.
Health Service Journal (1994a) 'NHS beats private hospitals to work', *Health Service Journal*, 14 April: 9.

Health Service Journal (1994b) 'Tax perks would "get private firms into NHS"', *Health Service Journal*, 28 April: 6.

Health Service Journal (1996) Back to square one', *Health Service Journal*, 25 January: 1.

Heginbotham C. (1992) 'Rationing', *British Medical Journal*, **34**: 496–7.

Henderson V. (1966) *The Nature of Nursing*, London, Collier Macmillan.

Henwood M. and Wistow G. (1995) 'The tasks in hand', *Health Service Journal*, 13 April: 24–5.

Hern J.E.C. (1994) 'Merit awards – the case for change', *British Medical Journal*, **308**: 973–4.

Higgins J. (1988) *The Business of Medicine: Private Health Care in Britain*, London, Macmillan Education.

Higgins J. and Ruddle S. (1991) 'Waiting for a better alternative', *Health Service Journal*, 11 July: 18–19.

Hoggett P. (1991) A new management in the public sector, *Policy and Politics*, **19**(4): 243–56.

Holmes S. (1994) 'Development of the cardiac surgeon's assistant', *British Journal of Nursing*, **3**: 204–10.

Honigsbaum F. (1979) *The Division in British Medicine*, London, Kogan Page.

Hopkins S. (1996) 'Junior doctors' hours and the expanding role of the nurse', *Nursing Times*, **92**(14): 35–6.

Hopton J.L. and Dlugolecka M. (1995) 'Need and demand for primary health care: a comparative survey approach', *British Medical Journal*, **310**: 1369–73.

Hudson B. (1992) 'Community care planning: incrementalism to rationalism?' *Social Policy and Administration*, **25**(3): 185–200.

Hudson B. (1993) 'The Icarus effect', *Health Service Journal*, 18 November: 27–9.

Hudson B. (1995a) 'Joint commissioning: organisational revolution or misplaced enthusiasm', *Policy and Politics*, **23**(3): 233–49.

Hudson B. (1995b) 'Could do better', *Health Service Journal*, 30 November: 30–1.

Hudson B. (1995c) 'Nothing ventured, nothing gained', *Health Service Journal*, 26 October: 26–7.

Hudson B. (1996) 'Health, housing, hiatus', *Health Service Journal*, 20 June: 29–30.

Hughes D. and Griffiths L. (1996) '"But if you look at the coronary anatomy": risk and rationing in cardiac surgery', *Sociology of Health and Illness*, **18**(2): 172–97.

Humphreys J. and Davis K. (1995) ‘Quality assurance for contracting of education: a delegated system involving consortia of British NHS trusts’, *Journal of Advanced Nursing*, **21**: 537–43.

Hunter D. (1993) *Rationing Dilemmas in Health Care*, London, National Association of Health Authorities and Trusts.

Hunter D.J. (1991a) ‘Pain of going public’, *Health Service Journal,* 29 August: 20.

Hunter D.J. (1991b) ‘Managing medicine: a response to the “crisis”’, *Social Science and Medicine*, **32**(4): 441–8.

Hunter H. (1995) ‘Calculated snub’, *Health Service Journal*, 8 June: 11.

Huntington J. (1994) ‘Bottom of the class?’ *Health Service Journal*, 8 September: 22–3.

Institute of Health Services Management (1990) *Models of Clinical Management*, London, IHSM.

Isaacs A. (1993) ‘Impact of the EC on medical manpower in the United Kingdom’, *British Hospital Management*, 36–43.

Johnson N. (1987) *The Welfare State in Transition: The Theory and Practice of Welfare Pluralism*, Brighton, Harvester Press.

Johnson N. (1989) ‘The privatisation of welfare’, *Social Policy and Administration*, **23**(1): 17–30.

Joint Committee on Higher Medical Training (1992) *Training Handbook*, London, JCHMT.

Jowett S., Walton K. and Payne S. (1994) *Challenges and Change in Nurse Education: A Study of the Implementation of Project 2000*, Slough, National Foundation for Educational Research.

Judge K. and Benzeval M. (1991) ‘A formula for funding’, *Health Service Journal*, 2 May: 20–1.

Kendrick T., Sibbald B., Burns T. and Freeling P. (1991) ‘The role of GPs in the care of long-term mentally ill patients’, *British Medical Journal*, **302**(6775): 508.

Kennedy P. (1990) ‘A better way than clinical directorates’, *Health Services Management*, **86**(5): 211–15.

Klein R. (1989) *The Politics of the NHS*, London, Longman.

Klein R. (1991) ‘On the Oregon trail: rationing health care’, *British Medical Journal*, **302**: 1–2.

Klein R. (1992) ‘Warning signals from Oregon’, *British Medical Journal*, **304**: 1457–8.

Klein R. (1995) ‘Big bang health care reform – does it work?: the case of Britain’s 1991 National Health Service reforms’, *The Millbank Quarterly*, **73**(3): 301–37.

Labour Party (1994) Gordon Brown, Robin Cook and John Prescott, *Financing Infrastructure Investment: Promoting a Partnership between Public and Private Finance*, joint consultative paper prepared for the Labour Finance and Industry Group symposium on public–private finance, London, Labour Party.

Laing and Buisson (1995) *Laing's Review of Private Healthcare 1995*, London, Laing and Buisson Publications.

Laing and Buisson (1996) *Laing's Review of Private Healthcare 1996*, London, Laing and Buisson Publications.

Langham S., Gillam S. and Thorogood M. (1995) 'The carrot, the stick and the general practitioner: how have changes in financial incentives affected health promotion activity in general practice?' *British Journal of General Practice*, December: 665–8.

Leese B. and Bosanquet N. (1995) 'Family doctors and change in practice strategy since 1986', *British Medical Journal*, **310**: 705–8.

Le Grand J. (1991) 'Quasi-markets and social policy', *Economic Journal*, **101**(1): 256–67.

Le Grand J. and Bartlett W. (1993) 'Introduction' in Le Grand J. and Bartlett W. (eds) *Quasi-Markets and Social Policy*, London, Macmillan.

Letwin O. and Redwood J. (1988) *Britain's Biggest Enterprise: Ideas for Reform of the NHS*, London, Centre for Policy Studies.

Limb M. (1993) 'Scottish Office slammed for alleged infertility U-turn', *Health Service Journal*, 25 March: 8.

London Health Planning Consortium (1981) *Primary Health Care in London* (Acheson Report), London, DHSS.

Long R. and Salter B. (1994) 'Legal confusion and political control', *Health Service Journal*, 5 May: 18–20.

Lowry S. (1993) *Medical Education*, London, BMJ Publishing Group.

Lowy A., Brazier J., Fall M. *et al.* (1993) 'Minor surgery by general practitioners under the 1990 contract: effects on hospital workload', *British Medical Journal*, **307**: 413–7.

Macara A.W. (1994) 'Reforming the NHS reforms', *British Medical Journal*, **308**: 848–49.

Marshall T.H. (1950) *Citizenship and Social Class*, Cambridge, Cambridge University Press.

Mawhinney B. (1994) *Medical Staffing Policies: A Time for Change*, EL(94)13, London, HMSO.

Maxwell R.J. (1974) *Health Care: The Growing Dilemma*, New York, McKinsey and Co.

Maynard A. (1989) 'Pitfalls in the plans', *Health Service Journal*, 23 February: 238.

Maynard A. (1995) 'Are they barking mad?', *Health Service Journal*, 5 October: 21.

McBride G. (1990) 'Rationing health care in Oregon', *British Medical Journal*, **301**: 355–66.

McGregor G. (1990) 'Privatisation on parade', *Health Service Journal*, 3 May: 670.

McPherson K., Strong P.M., Epstein A. and Jones L. (1981) 'Regional variations in the use of common surgical procedures, within and between England and Wales', *Social Science and Medicine*, **15A**: 273–8.

Mechanic D. (1995) 'Dilemmas in rationing health care services: the case for implicit rationing', *British Medical Journal*, **310**: 1655–9.

Medical Manpower Standing Advisory Committee (1992) *Planning the Medical Workforce*, London, Department of Health.

Medical Workforce Standing Advisory Committee (1995) *Planning the Medical Workforce,* second report, London, Department of Health.

Medway NHS Trust (1994) *Contract for Postgraduate Medical and Dental Education*, Medway NHS Trust.

Melia K. (1987) *Learning and Working: The Occupational Socialisation of Nurses*, London, Tavistock.

Mental Health Foundation (1994) *Creating Community Care: Report of the Mental Health Foundation Inquiry into Community Care for People with Severe Mental Illness*, London, Mental Health Foundation.

Merrison Report (1975) *Report of the Committee of Inquiry into the Regulation of the Medical Profession*, (Chairman: Sir Alec Merrison), Cmnd 6018, London, HMSO.

Merry P. (1990) 'Sprited defence of community health doctors', *British Medical Journal*, **300**: 1591.

Millar B. (1991) 'Clinicians as managers: medics make their minds up', *Health Service Journal*, 21 February: 17.

Ministry of Health (1966) *Report of the Committee on Senior Nursing Staff*, Salmon Report, London, HMSO.

Mishra R. (1984) *The Welfare State in Crisis*, Brighton, Wheatsheaf.

Mitchell J.R.A. (1984) 'Is nursing any business of doctors? a simple guide to the nursing process', *British Medical Journal*, **288**: 216–19.

Mohan J. (1986) 'Private medical care and the British Conservative government: what price independence?', *Journal of Social Policy*, **15**(3): 337–60.

Mohan J. (1992) 'Privatisation in the British health sector: a challenge to the NHS?' in Gabe J., Calnan M. and Bury M. (eds) *The Sociology of the Health Service*, London, Routledge, pp. 36–57.

Mohan J. and Woods K. (1985) 'Restructuring health care: the social geography of public and private health care under the British Conservative Government', *International Journal of Health Services*, **15**: 197–215.

Monopolies and Mergers Commission (1993) *Private Medical Services: A Report on Agreements and Practices Relating to Charges for the Supply of Private Medical Services by NHS Consultants*, London, HMSO.

Montgomery J. (1992) 'Doctors' handmaidens: the legal contribution' in McVeigh S. and Wheeler S. (eds) *Law, Health and Medical Regulation*, Aldershot, Dartmouth.

Moore W. (1992a) 'Public health chief's drug call sparks off row over rationing', *Health Service Journal*, 13 February: 6.

Moore W. (1992b) 'May the force be with you', *Health Service Journal*, 24 September: 12.

Moore W. (1995) 'Is doctors' power shrinking?' *Health Service Journal*, 9 November: 24–7.

Moran M. and Wood B. (1993) *States, Regulation and the Medical Profession*, Buckingham, Open University Press.

Morrell D.C., Gage H.G. and Robinson N.A. (1971) 'Referral to hospital by general practitioners', *Journal of the Royal College of General Practice*, **21**: 77–85.

Morris F., Head S. and Holkar V. (1989) 'The nurse practitioner: help in clarifying clinical and educational activities in A and E departments', *Health Trends*, **21**: 124–6.

Morrison I. and Smith R. (1994) 'The future of medicine', *British Medical Journal*, **309**: 1099–100.

National Association of Health Authorities and Trusts (1995) *A Health Authority Perspective on Community Care: A Survey of Special Transitional Grant Agreements 1995/6*, Birmingham, NAHAT.

National Audit Office (1988) *Management of the Family Practitioner Service*, HC498, London, HMSO.

National Audit Office (1992) *Nursing Education: Implementation of Project 2000 in England*, HC291, London, HMSO.

National Audit Office (1993) *Income Generation in the NHS*, London, HMSO.

National Audit Office (1996) *Health of the Nation: A Progress Report*, London, HMSO.

National Health Service Executive (1992a) *Local Voices: The Views of Local People in Purchasing for Health*, Leeds, NHSE.

National Health Service Executive (1992b) *The Funding of Hospital Medical and Dental Training Grade Posts*, EL(92)63, Leeds NHSE.

National Health Service Executive (1993a) *Improving Clinical Effectiveness*, EL(93)115, Leeds, NHSE.

National Health Service Executive (1993b) *Managing Activity and Change Through Contracts*, EL(93)10, Leeds, NHSE.

National Health Service Executive (1993c) *Medical Advice to Purchasers*, EL(93)60, Leeds, NHSE.
National Health Service Executive (1993d) *The Use of Private Capital in the NHS*, FDL(93)03, Leeds, NHSE.
National Health Service Executive (1993e) *Private Finance in the NHS: Approval Procedures*, FDL(93)33, Leeds, NHSE.
National Health Service Executive (1993f) *Private Finance Guidance on Leasing*, FDL(93)47, Leeds, NHSE.
National Health Service Executive (1993g) *Guidance for Financial Institutions and Others Trading with NHS Trusts*, FDL(93)51, Leeds, NHSE.
National Health Service Executive (1994a) *Code of Conduct*, London, Department of Health.
National Health Service Executive (1994b) *Code of Accountability*, London, Department of Health.
National Health Service Executive (1994c) *Codes of Conduct and Accountability: Guidance*, EL(94)40, Leeds, NHSE.
National Health Service Executive (1994d) *Developing NHS purchasing and GP Fundholding. Towards a Primary Care Led NHS*, Leeds, NHSE.
National Health Service Executive (1994e) *Developing NHS Purchasing and GP Fundholders*, EL(94)79, Leeds, NHSE.
National Health Service Executive (1994f) *Improving the Effectiveness of the NHS*, EL(94)74, Leeds, NHSE.
National Health Service Executive (1994g) *Towards A Primary Care Led NHS: An Accountability Framework for GP Fundholding*, EL(94)92, Leeds, NHSE.
National Health Service Executive (1994h) *Capital Investment in the NHS – The Capital Investment Manual*, HSG(94)31, Leeds, NHSE.
National Health Service Executive (1995a) *Code of Practice on Openness in the NHS*, Leeds, NHSE.
National Health Service Executive (1995b) *Acting on Complaints, the Government's Proposals in Response to 'Being Heard'*, Leeds, NHSE.
National Health Service Executive (1995c) *Priorities and Planning: Guidance for the NHS*, EL(95)68, Leeds, NHSE.
National Health Service Executive (1995d) *Education and Training in the New NHS*, EL(95)27, Leeds, NHSE.
National Health Service Executive (1995e) *Private Finance and Capital Investment Projects*, HSG(95)15, Leeds, NHSE.
National Health Service Executive (1995f) *Information Management and Technology (IM and T) Procurement and Private Finance*, HSG(95)48, Leeds, NHSE.

National Health Service Management Executive (1989a) *The Role of District Health Authorities – Analysis of Issues*, London, Department of Health.

National Health Service Management Executive (1990a) *NHS Trusts: A Working Guide*, London, HMSO.

National Health Service Management Executive (1991a) *Priorities and Planning Guidance for the NHS for 1992/93*, EL(91)103, Leeds, NHSME.

National Health Service Management Executive (1991b) *Moving Forward: Needs, Services and Contracts*, London, Department of Health.

National Health Service Management Executive (1991c) *Assessing Health Care Needs*, London, Department of Health.

National Health Service Management Executive (1991d) *Purchasing Intelligence*, London, Department of Health.

National Health Service Management Executive (1991e) *Integrating Primary and Secondary Health Care*, London, Department of Health.

National Health Service Management Executive (1991f) *Working for Patients. Postgraduate and Continuing Medical Education*, Leeds, NHSME.

National Health Service Management Executive (1991g) *Hours of Work of Doctors in Training: The New Deal*, EL(91)82, Leeds, NHSME.

National Health Service Management Executive (1991h) *Appointments of Consultant Medical and Dental Staff to NHS Trusts*, TEL(91)2, Leeds, NHSME.

National Health Service Management Executive (1992) *Withdrawal of Guidance on the Extended Role of the Nurse*, EL(92)38, PL/CNO(92)4, Leeds, NHSME.

National Health Service Training Authority (1987) *Managing with Doctors: Working Together*. Templeton Series on District General Manager, Issue Study no. 5, London.

Newton V. (1996) 'Care in pre-admission clinics', *Nursing Times*, 3 January, **92**(1): 27.

No Turning Back Group (1990) *Choice and Responsibility: The Enabling State*, London, Conservative Political Centre.

Nursing Times (1995) 'ENB approves new high-tech training', *Nursing Times*, 7 June, **91**(23): 9.

Offe K. (1983) *Contradictions of the Welfare State*, London, Hutchinson.

Office of Health Economics (1995) *Compendium of Health Statistics*, London, OHE.

Packwood T., Buxton M. and Keen J. (1990) 'Resource management in the National Health Service: a first case history', *Policy and Politics*, **18**(4): 245–55.

Pallot P. (1994) 'NHS trust manager attacked for saying patients come third', *Telegraph*, 14 November: 7.

Papadakis E. and Taylor-Gooby P. (1987) *The Private Provision of Public Welfare: State, Market and Community*, Brighton, Wheatsheaf.

Pearson A. (1988) *Therapeutic Nursing: An Evaluation of an Experimental Nursing Unit in the British NHS*, Oxford, Burford and Oxford Nurse Development Units.

Pearson A. (1992) *Nursing at Burford: A Story of Change*, London, Scutari Press.

Pearson A., Punton S. and Durant I. (1992) *Nursing Beds: An Evaluation of the Effects of Therapeutic Nursing*, London, Scutari Press.

Pettigrew A., McKee L. and Ferlie E. (1988) 'Understanding change in the NHS', *Public Administration*, **66**(3): 297–317.

Pickersgill F. (1995) 'A natural extension?' *Nursing Times*, 26 July, **91**(30): 24–7.

Pinker R. (1992) 'Making sense of the mixed economy of welfare', *Social Policy and Administration*, **26**(4): 273–84.

Pope C. (1992) 'Cutting queues or cutting corners: waiting lists and the 1990 NHS reforms', *British Medical Journal*, **305**: 577–9.

Porter R. (1987) *Disease, Medicine and Society in England 1550–1860*, London, Macmillan.

Potter T. (1990) 'A real way forward in A and E: developing the nurse practitioner role', *Professional Nurse*, **5**(11): 586–8.

Ranson S. and Stewart J. (1989) 'Citizenship and government: the challenge for management in the public domain', *Political Studies*, **37**: 5–24.

Rayner G. (1986) 'Health care as business? The emergence of a commercial hospital sector in Britain', *Policy and Politics*, **14**(4): 439–59.

Read S. and George M. (1994) 'Nurse practitioners in accident and emergency departments: reflections on a pilot study', *Journal of Advanced Nursing*, **19**(4): 705–16.

Read S. and Graves K. (1994) *Reduction of Junior Doctor Hours in the Trent Region. The Nursing Contribution*, Trent RHA, NHSE.

Read S., Jones N. and Williams B. (1992) 'Nurse practitioners in A and E Departments: what do they do?, *British Medical Journal*, **305**: 1466–70.

Redmayne S. (1992) 'Skin deep', *Health Service Journal*, 22 October: 28–9.

Redwood J. (1988) *In Sickness and in Health: Managing Change in the NHS*, London, Centre for Policy Studies.

Rees A.M. (1972) 'Access to the personal health and welfare services', *Social and Economic Administration*, **6**(1): 38–42.

Relman R. (1990) 'The trouble with rationing', *New England Journal of Medicine*, 323: 911–13.

Richards J. and Robinson R. (1994) 'Allied powers', *Health Service Journal*, 15 September: 24–5.

Richards P. (1992) 'Educational improvement of the pre-registration period of general clinical training', *British Medical Journal*, **304**: 625–7.

Rimlinger G.V. (1971) *Welfare Policy and Industrialisation in Europe, America and Russia*, New York, John Wiley.

Rink E., Hilton S., Szczepura A. *et al.* (1993) 'Impact of introducing near patient testing for standard investigations in general practice', *British Medical Journal*, **307**: 775–8.

Robinson K. (1992) 'The nursing workforce: aspects of inequality' in Robinson J., Gray A. and Elkan R. (eds) *Policy Issues in Nursing*, Buckingham, Open University Press, pp. 24–37.

Roland M.O., Bartholomew J., Morrell D.C. *et al.* (1990) 'Understanding hospital referral rates: a user's guide', *British Medical Journal*, **301**: 98–102.

Rose R. (1986) 'Common goals but different roles: the state's contribution to the welfare mix' in Rose R. and Shiratori R. (eds) *The Welfare State in East and West*, New York/Oxford, Oxford University Press.

Royal College of General Practitioners (1992) *Response to 'Caring For People'*, Cm 849.

Royal College of Nursing (1981) *Towards Standards*, London, RCN.

Royal College of Nursing (1985) *The Education of Nurses: A New Dispensation,* (Chair: Professor H. Judge), London, Royal College of Nursing.

Royal College of Physicians of London (1989) *Medical Audit: A First Report, What, Why and How?* London, RCP of London.

Royal College of Physicians (1995) *Setting Priorities in the NHS. A Framework for Decision Making*, London, RCP.

Royal College of Surgeons of England (1988) Commission on the Provision of Surgical Services, *Report of the Working Party on the Composition of a Surgical Team – General Surgery, Orthopaedics and Otolaryngology*, London, RCS.

Royal College of Surgeons of England (1989) *Guidelines to Clinical Audit in Surgical Practice*, London, RCS.

Royal Commission on the Law Relating to Mental Illness and Mental Deficiency 1954–1957 (1957) *Report*, Cmnd 169, London, HMSO.

Royce R. (1995) 'Creative tensions', *Health Service Journal*, 6 July: 26.

Salomans Centre (1995) *Developing the Role and Purpose of NHS Boards*, Tunbridge Wells, Salomans Centre.

Salter B. (1991a) 'A difficult choice', *Health Services Management*, **4**(3): 111–13.

Salter B. (1991b) 'Demand and fallacy', *Health Service Journal*, 5 December: 19.

Salter B. (1992a) 'Heart of the matter', *Health Service Journal*, 1 October: 30–1.

Salter B. (1993a) 'Public image limited', *Health Service Journal*, 15 July: 28–9.

Salter B. (1993b) 'The politics of purchasing in the National Health Service', *Policy and Politics*, **21**(3): 171–84.

Salter B. (1994a) 'The politics of community care: social rights and welfare limits', *Policy and Politics*, **22**(2): 119–31.

Salter B. (1994b) 'Change in the British National Health Service, policy paradox and the rationing issue', *International Journal of Health Services*, **24**(1): 45–72.

Salter B. and Douglas G. (1994) 'Private money and public health: managing the risks', *Health Services Management*, April: 10–11.

Salter B. and Salter C. (1993) 'Theatre of the absurd', *Health Service Journal*, 11 November: 30–1.

Salter B. and Snee N. (1997) 'Power dressing', *Health Service Journal*, 13 February: 30–1.

Salvage J. (1992) 'The new nursing: empowering patients or empowering nurses?' in Robinson J., Gray A. and Elkan R. (eds) *Policy Issues in Nursing*, Buckingham, Open University Press, pp. 10–23.

Saper R. and Laing W. (1995) 'Age of uncertainty', *Health Service Journal*, 20 October: 22–3.

Scrivens E. (1987) 'The management of clinicians in the NHS', *Social Policy and Adminstration*, **22**(1): 22–34.

Seebohm Report (1968) *Local Authority and Allied Social Services*, London, HMSO.

Seccombe I. and Smith G. (1996) *In the Balance: Registered Nurse Supply and Demand*, Brighton, Institute For Employment Studies.

Sheldon T. and Carr-Hill R. (1991a) 'Right approach, wrong market', *Health Service Journal*, 8 August: 24–5.

Sheldon T. and Carr-Hill R. (1991b) 'Equity and efficiency', *Health Service Journal*, 25 July: 18–19, 22–3.

Sheldon T. and Carr-Hill R. (1991c) 'Measure for measure', *Health Service Journal*, 1 August: 22–3.

Sheldon T., Smith P., Borowitz M., Martin S. and Carr-Hill R. (1994) 'Attempt at deriving a formula for setting general practitioner fundholding budgets', *British Medical Journal*, **309**: 1059–64.

Short J.A. (1995) 'Has nursing lost its way?' *British Medical Journal*, **311**: 303–4.

Smith J. (1993) 'Newcastle: if it doesn't work here, it can't work anywhere', *British Medical Journal*, **306**: 566–9.

Smith R. (1989a) 'Profile of the GMC: 1978 and all that', *British Medical Journal*, **298**: 1297–300.

Smith R. (1989b) 'Discipline I: the hordes at the gates', *British Medical Journal*, **298**: 1502–05.

Smith R. (1991) 'Rationing: the search for sunlight', *British Medical Journal*, **303**: 1561–2.

Smith R. (1992) 'The GMC on performance', *British Medical Journal*, **304**: 1257–8.

Smith R. (1994) 'Medicine's core values', *British Medical Journal*, **309**: 1247–8.

Smith R. (1995a) 'Rationing: the debate we have to have', *British Medical Journal*, **310**: 686.

Smith R. (1995b) 'The future of the GMC: an interview with Donald Irvine, the new president', *British Medical Journal*, **310**: 1515–18.

Social Services Committee of the House of Commons (1985) *Community Care*, second report, Session 1984–85, HC13–I, London, HMSO.

Social Services Committee of the House of Commons (1988) *Resourcing the National Health Service: Short Term Issues*, fourth report, Session 1987–88, HC264–I, London, HMSO.

Society for Social Medicine (1990) 33rd Annual Scientific Meeting, 'The ethics of resource allocation', Proceedings of a symposium held at the University of Manchester, *Journal of Epidemiology and Community Health*, **44**: 187–90.

Spry C. (1990) 'Clinical directorates: a management point of view' in Costain D. (ed.) *The Future of Acute Services: Doctors as Managers*, London, King's Fund Centre for Health Service Development.

Stacey M. (1984) 'The General Medical Council and professional accountability', *Public Policy and Administration*, **4**(1): 12–27.

Standing Committee on Postgraduate and Continuing Medical Education (1990) *An Assessment of NHS Expenditure on Postgraduate Medical Education in England 1988/89*, London, SCOPME.

Standing Medical Advisory Committee and Standing Nursing and Midwifery Committee (1981) *The Primary Health Care Team*, London, (Harding Report).

Starr P. (1982) *The Social Transformation of American Medicine*, New York, Basic Books.

Stevens A. and Gabbay J. (1991) 'Needs assessment needs assessment', *Health Trends*, **23**(1): 20–3.

Stewart-Brown S., Surender R., Bradlow J. *et al.* (1995) 'The effects of fundholding in general practice on prescribing habits three years after introduction of the scheme', *British Medical Journal*, **311**: 1543–7.

Stilwell B. (1987) 'A nurse practitioner in general practice: working style and pattern of consultations', *Journal of Royal College of General Practitioners*, **37**: 154–7.

Stock J., Seccombe I. and Patch A. (1994) *Opening the Door: Employment, Prospects and Morale of Newly Qualified Nurses*, London, Institute for Employment Studies and Royal College of Nursing.

Strachan S. (1991) *Making it Happen: The Role of the Authority Chief Executive*, London, King's Fund.

Taylor D. (1991) 'Funding Family Health Services', *British Medical Journal*, **303**: 562–4.

Taylor-Gooby P. (1996) 'The future of health care in six European countries: the view of policy elites', *International Journal of Health Services*, **26**(2): 203–19.

Taylor-Gooby P. and Lawson R. (1993) *Markets and Managers, New Issues in the Delivery of Welfare*, Buckingham, Open University Press.

Thompson D. (1987) 'Coalitions and conflict in the NHS: some implications for general management', *Sociology of Health and Illness*, **9**(2): 127–53.

Thornicroft G., Ward P. and James S. (1993) 'Care management and mental health', *British Medical Journal*, **306**: 768–71.

Thwaites Prof. Sir Bryan (1987) *The NHS, the End of the Rainbow*, The University of Southampton, Institute of Health Policy Studies, The Foundation Lecture, May.

Tomlin Z. (1990) 'No manager is an island – nor is any doctor', *Health Service Journal*, 20 December: 13.

Treasury Committee of the House of Commons (1996) *The Private Finance Initiative*, sixth report, House of Commons, Session 1995–96, HC146.

Trnobranski (1994) 'Nurse practitioner: redefining the role of the community nurse?', *Journal of Advanced Nursing*, **19**(1): 134–9.

Turner S. (1995) 'NHSE study shows doctors are hostile to management', *British Medical Association, News Review*, December: 13.

United Kingdom Central Council for Nursing (1986a) *Project 2000, A New Preparation for Practice*, London, UKCC.

United Kingdom Central Council for Nursing (1986b) *Administration of Medicine*, London, UKCC.

United Kingdom Central Council for Nursing (1987) *Project 2000: The Final Proposals*, London, UKCC.

United Kingdom Central Council for Nursing (1989) *Exercising Accountability,* London, UKCC.

United Kingdom Central Council for Nursing (1992a) *The Scope of Professional Practice*, London, UKCC.

United Kingdom Central Council for Nursing (1992b) *Code of Professional Conduct,* London, UKCC.

United Kingdom Central Council for Nursing (1995) *PREP and You – Implementation of the UKCCs Standards for Post-Registration Education and Practice*, London, UKCC.

Van Steenbergen B. (1994) 'The condition of citizenship: an introduction' in Van Steenbergen B. (ed.) *The Condition of Citizenship*, London, Sage.

Walby S., Greenwell J., Mackay L. and Soothill K. (1994) *Medicine and Nursing*, London, Sage.

Walker A. (1988) 'Tendering care', *New Society*, **83**(1308): 18–19.

Ward S. (1994) 'Education for life', *British Medical Association, News Review*, September: 18–19.

Warden J. (1995a) 'NHS managers to go in new purge by Dorrell', *British Medical Journal*, **311**: 1591.

Warden J. (1995b) 'Britain seeks more home grown doctors', *British Medical Journal*, **311**: 9.

Warner N. (1995) *Community Care: Just a Fairy Tale?* London, Carers National Association.

Waters J. (1995) 'Highland clearances', *Health Service Journal*, 16 November: 13.

Weisbrod B. (1988) *The Non–profit Economy*, Cambridge, Cambridge University Press.

Willetts D. (1993) *The Opportunities for Private Funding in the NHS*, occasional paper, London, Social Market Foundation.

West C. (1992) 'A general manager's view of contemporary nursing issues' in Robinson J., Gray A. and Elkan R. (eds) *Policy Issues in Nursing*, Buckingham, Open University Press.

West R. (1993) 'Joining the queue: demand and decision making' in Frankel S. and West R. *Rationing and Rationality in the NHS. The Persistence of Waiting Lists*, Basingstoke, Macmillan, pp. 47–66.

White M. (1995) 'Nocturnal ramblings over GPs' night calls', *Health Service Journal*, 20 July: 22.

Whynes D.K. (1992) 'The growth of UK public health expenditure', *Social Policy and Administration*, **26**(4): 285–304.

Whynes D.K., Baines D.L. and Tolley K.H. (1995) 'GP fundholding and the costs of prescribing', *Journal of Public Health Medicine*, **17**(3): 323–9.

Wichowski H.C. (1994) 'Professional uncertainty: nurses in the technologically intense arena', *Journal of Advanced Nursing*, **19**(6): 1162–7.

Wilkin D. and Smith A. (1988) 'Explaining variation in general practitioner referrals to hospital', *Family Practitioner*, **4**: 160–9.

Willetts D. (1993) *The Opportunities for Private Funding in the NHS*, occasional paper, London, Social Market Foundation.

Williams A. (1985) 'Economies of coronary artery bypass grafting', *British Medical Journal*, **291**: 326–9.

Williams A. (1988) 'Health economics: the end of clinical freedom', *British Medical Journal*, **297**: 1183–6.

Williamson C. (1995) 'Spice of life', *Health Service Journal*, 23 March: 28–9.

Wilson D.H. (1993) 'Education and training of pre-registration house officers: the consultants' viewpoint', *British Medical Journal*, **306**: 194–6.

Wistow G. (1995) 'Coming apart at the seams', *Health Service Journal*, 2 March: 25.

Wistow G., Hardy B. and Leedham I. (1993) 'Planning blight', *Health Service Journal*, 18 February: 22–4.

Wistow G., Knapp M., Hardy B. and Allen C. (1992) 'From providing to enabling, local authorities and the mixed economy of care', *Public Administration*, **70**: 25–45.

Witz A. (1994) 'The challenge to nursing' in Gabe J., Kelleher D. and Williams G. (eds) *Challenging Medicine*, London, Routledge.

Woodhead A. (1996) 'An extra-special relationship', *Health Service Journal*, 4 January: 26–7.

Working Group on Specialist Medical Training (1993) *Hospital Doctors: Training for the Future*, London (Calman Report).

Wright T. (1996) 'In on the act', *Health Service Journal*, 16 May: 12.

Young A. (1986) *Evaluating Management Budgeting in the NHS*, Glasgow, Young Consultants.

Yura H. and Walsh M. (1978) *The Nursing Process*, New York, Appleton-Century-Crofts.

Index

D

E

F

G

N

Q

R